A SHORT INTRODUCTION TO
COUNSELLING

Sally Aldridge

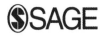SAGE

Los Angeles | London | New Delhi
Singapore | Washington DC

080771
361.323 ALD
cnc

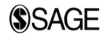

Los Angeles | London | New Delhi
Singapore | Washington DC

SAGE Publications Ltd
1 Oliver's Yard
55 City Road
London EC1Y 1SP

SAGE Publications Inc.
2455 Teller Road
Thousand Oaks, California 91320

SAGE Publications India Pvt Ltd
B 1/I 1 Mohan Cooperative Industrial Area
Mathura Road
New Delhi 110 044

SAGE Publications Asia-Pacific Pte Ltd
3 Church Street
#10-04 Samsung Hub
Singapore 049483

Editor: Kate Wharton
Editorial assistant: Laura Walmsley
Production editor: Rachel Burrows
Copyeditor: Jill Birch
Proofreader: Anna Gilding
Indexer: Avril Ehrlich
Marketing manager: Tamara Navaratnam
Cover design: Lisa Harper
Typeset by: C&M Digitals (P) Ltd, Chennai, India
Printed in Great Britain by Henry Ling Limited at
The Dorset Press, Dorchester, DT1 1HD

Library of Congress Control Number: 2013944555

British Library Cataloguing in Publication data

A catalogue record for this book is available from
the British Library

MIX
Paper from
responsible sources
FSC
www.fsc.org   FSC™ C013985

ISBN 978-1-4462-5256-7
ISBN 978-1-4462-5257-4 (pbk)

To Clive for his patience over lost weekends
and evenings

To BACP for the best job I've ever had

CONTENTS

ABOUT THE AUTHOR

Dr Sally Aldridge has been actively involved in counselling since qualifying as a counsellor at the University of Keele. As is the case with many counsellors, this is a second career; the first was as a teacher of African History in Zambia. Sally worked as a student counsellor, supervisor and trainer before joining BACP as a full time member of staff responsible for the accreditation schemes in 1999. Sally had previously been involved with BACP as a volunteer in the accreditation schemes and an elected member of the Management Committee. She is a Fellow of BACP.

Sally sees her own career developing in parallel with the development of BACP and counselling in the United Kingdom. This led her to a doctorate in the development of counselling in 2011 titled *Counselling – an insecure profession? A historical and sociological analysis*. Previous publications include, *Counselling Skills in Context* (Hodder & Stoughton, 2001) and *The Peoples of Zambia* (Heinemann Educational Books, 1978).

Sally has been a member of many national projects related to counselling and psychotherapy: the development of National Occupational Standards for the Psychological Therapies, the Improving Access to Psychological Therapies Workforce and Education and Training Groups, New Ways of Working for Psychological Therapists, the Health Professions Council's Professional Liaison Group for the statutory regulation of psychotherapy and counselling and the Quality Assurance Agency Benchmark Development Group for Counselling and Psychotherapy. She is currently a member of the Steering Group for the expansion of psychological therapy in Northern Ireland.

In order to stay calm Sally runs and in 2012 became a 'Compleat Runner' in her local league by completing all 22 races in 10 months.

1 WHAT IS COUNSELLING?

INTRODUCTION

> Taxi driver to passenger: 'What do you do?'
> Passenger: 'I'm a counsellor.'
> Taxi driver: 'A town councillor?'
> Passenger: 'No. You've heard of Relate, Marriage Guidance Counselling? Well like that but for all sorts of problems.'

This dialogue captures some of the difficulties counselling has in defining itself. One of the problems is that the term 'counselling' is used in contexts other than the therapeutic: a debt counsellor gives you debt advice and help with employment and consumer law. Google 'counsellor' and the fourth and fifth entries are for 'travel counsellors' who will sell you a holiday. Members of the public seeking counselling know the difference and are very unlikely to ask you about the thermal properties of new windows.

This chapter addresses the question 'What is counselling?' from a number of perspectives, starting with a range of definitions of counselling and the terms in common use to describe the therapies. There is a brief account of the origins and development of counselling that also traces the separation of counselling from other forms of helping such as guidance and befriending in the 1990s. The chapter then looks at some of the different views of the nature and purpose of counselling within the field and considers the social and political dimensions of counselling. Finally it describes the positions held on the difference between counselling and psychotherapy. Throughout, this book is about working with individuals rather than couples or groups.

Counselling has been a feature of everyday life since the second half of the twentieth century and yet even when experts are employed to carry out the task, they find that 'the counselling sector is difficult to define' (ENTO 2008: 29). Despite, or perhaps because of this, it is estimated that there are 100,000 people delivering therapy in the United Kingdom (Mental Health Foundation, Mind et al. 2006), the majority describing what they do as counselling.

DEFINITIONS OF COUNSELLING

There are several definitions of counselling in circulation. Some are exclusive to counselling, some are inclusive of all the talking therapies and some seek to differentiate between the various talking therapies. Most of the definitions of counselling below are written by professional organisations and reflect the views of their members; or by organisations and government agencies and reflect the services on offer. The first two British Association for Counselling/British Association for Counselling and Psychotherapy (BAC/BACP) definitions from 1978 and 2013 illustrate the development of counselling during that time.

1978 Definition by the Standing Conference for the Advancement of Counselling/British Association for Counselling

'Counselling takes place when one person accepts responsibility for helping another to decide upon a course of action or to understand or change patterns of behaviour which distress, disturb or affect his social behaviour.' The definition continues to describe when counselling takes place and states that counselling may be 'incidental to the other functions of the professional' for example a teacher and pupil. It may be 'educational and vocational guidance, provided by a specialist service for particular problems or within voluntary agencies' (Standing Conference for the Advancement of Counselling 1978).

2013 BACP Definition One

> Counselling and psychotherapy are umbrella terms that cover a range of talking therapies. They are delivered by trained practitioners who work with people over a short or long term to help them bring about effective change or enhance their wellbeing.
>
> Therapy is time set aside by you and the therapist to look at what has brought you to therapy. This might include talking about life events (past and present), feelings, emotions, relationships, ways of thinking and patterns of behaviour. The therapist will do their best to help you to look at your issues, and to identify the right course of action for you, either to help you resolve your difficulties or help you find ways of coping. Talking about these things may take time, and will not necessarily all be included in one session. The number of sessions offered may be limited, and so it is best to ask about this in advance, for example, brief therapy or short term therapy might provide a maximum of 6, 8, 10 or 12 sessions. (www.bacp.co.uk/crs/Training/whatis counselling.php)

2013 BACP Definition Two

Counselling takes place when a counsellor sees a client in a private and confidential setting to explore a difficulty the client is having, distress they may be experiencing or perhaps their dissatisfaction with life, or loss of a sense of direction and purpose. It is always at the request of the client as no one can properly be 'sent' for counselling.

By listening attentively and patiently the counsellor can begin to perceive the difficulties from the client's point of view and can help them to see things more clearly, possibly from a different perspective. Counselling is a way of enabling choice or change or of reducing confusion. It does not involve giving advice or directing a client to take a particular course of action. Counsellors do not judge or exploit their clients in any way.

In the counselling sessions the client can explore various aspects of their life and feelings, talking about them freely and openly in a way that is rarely possible with friends or family. Bottled up feelings such as anger, anxiety, grief and embarrassment can become very intense and counselling offers an opportunity to explore them, with the possibility of making them easier to understand. The counsellor will encourage the expression of feelings and as a result of their training will be able to accept and reflect the client's problems without becoming burdened by them.

Acceptance and respect for the client are essentials for a counsellor and, as the relationship develops, so too does trust between the counsellor and client, enabling the client to look at many aspects of their life, their relationships and themselves which they may not have considered or been able to face before. The counsellor may help the client to examine in detail the behaviour or situations which are proving troublesome and to find an area where it would be possible to initiate some change as a start. The counsellor may help the client to look at the options open to them and help them to decide the best for them. (www.bacp.co.uk/crs/Training/whatiscounselling.php)

MIND (the mental health charity) Definition

Counselling provides a regular time and space for people to talk about their troubles and explore difficult feelings, in an environment that is dependable, free from intrusion and confidential. A counsellor should respect your viewpoint, while helping you to deal with specific problems, cope with crises, improve your relationships, or develop better ways of living. Despite the name, counsellors don't usually offer advice. Instead, they help you to gain insight into your feelings and behaviour and to change your behaviour, if necessary. They do this by listening to what you have to say and commenting on it from their particular professional perspective. The word 'counselling' covers a broad spectrum, from someone who is highly trained to someone who uses counselling skills (listening, reflecting back what you say, or clarifying) as part of another role, such as nursing. We use the term here to mean a talking therapy delivered by a trained professional. Sessions usually take place once a week. Making this regular commitment gives you a better chance of finding out why you are having difficulties. (Catty 2010)

United Kingdom Council for Psychotherapy's (UKCP) definition of psychotherapeutic counselling

Psychotherapeutic Counselling is distinguished from traditional counselling by its emphasis on the co-creation of an in-depth therapeutic relationship; wherein the suffering human being is viewed holistically, body, mind and soul and in the context of a concrete life situation and developmental stage. When training as a psychotherapeutic counsellor there is particular reference to establishing and maintaining the *therapeutic relationship*, which is the central factor in the work. (www.psychotherapy.org.uk/psychotherapeeutic brcounselling.html)

Royal College of Psychiatrists' definition

Counselling is a general term for exploring emotional problems by talking them through with a trained counsellor or therapist. The term covers a considerable range of approaches. In its simplest form, this can be supportive and sympathetic listening in the form of weekly sessions over a small number of weeks. This sort of counselling is suited to people with fundamentally healthy personalities who need help in addressing a current crisis in their life or relationships.

Some more experienced counsellors, who have had further training in any of a large range of theoretical approaches, work in a deeper way, and are able to help people with more complex problems. (www.rcpsych.ac.uk/workin psychiatry/faculties/medicalpsychotherapy/nhspsychologicaltreatment. aspx#counsel)

In all of these definitions counselling is a term used to describe a helping relationship. One person, 'the client', has an issue or a problem, something that he or she cannot deal with alone. The 'client' approaches the 'counsellor' for help in a formal confidential relationship. The purpose of this relationship is to help the 'client' address or deal better with his or her issues.

The client's definition of counselling

While most people seem to know what counselling is, when asked, there are few definitions of counselling written by clients. Those that exist derive from research and market research into what clients want from counselling. Clients want to be treated with respect, to be understood and helped to resolve problems. Counselling provides another person who is willing to help the client do that. Clients want a counselling relationship that treats them as individuals with acceptance and hope (Brainchild UK Ltd 2008).

A BACP-commissioned project with clients produced many images of their hopes for therapy – the one I remember is a blue velvet armchair with arms like wings. Several others showed journeys from dark places to the light (Forsythe and Corfino 2008: 28). These provide the clients' ideas of good counselling as being an empathic non-judgmental relationship; a process that will give hope and help people to feel better (Forsythe and Corfino 2008: 26). In summary it has proved almost impossible to come up with a definition that is boundaried, succinct and clear. There is not the same problem of definition with 'psychology', 'psychiatry' or 'psychotherapy'. There is a different problem for these groups – any word with 'psy' at the beginning is taken to imply mental illness (Forsythe and Corfino 2008).

THE TALKING OR PSYCHOLOGICAL THERAPIES

Counselling is one of the groups of occupations described as Talking Therapies and Psychological Therapies, together with psychiatry, clinical and counselling psychology and psychotherapy. Talking Therapies and Psychological Therapies are terms used in the literature of the Departments of Health of the four home countries and of charitable organisations dealing with mental health such as MIND. MIND, for example, uses the term 'talking treatments' and includes within this psychotherapy, counselling and therapy stating that,

> the terms 'talking treatment' or 'talking therapy' or 'psychological therapy'… cover treatments that you may know as
>
> - psychotherapy
> - counselling
> - therapy.

MIND also lists the titles a 'specially trained mental health professional' might work under:

- Counsellor
- Psychotherapist
- Psychologist
- Psychiatrist
- Therapist (www.mind.org.uk/mental_health_a-z/7972_making_sense_of_talking_treatments)

Some people see counselling as a non-professional activity, as an everyday relationship that does not require training, only human understanding and a willingness to help in dealing with another person's hurt and distress.

Others, see counselling as an equal partner with psychotherapy, psychology and psychoanalysis. Some in these professions regard counselling as a junior partner, dealing with simpler problems more quickly. Some commentators have presented counselling as the future hope for society, the replacement for organised religion and the extended family and as such an agent to support social cohesion (Halmos 1964; 1967). Counselling is seen as a response to the increased emphasis in society on the individual rather than the family or community. This has led to a number of views critical of the role of counselling. One view sees it as weakening the moral fibre of the population, making people into therapy junkies unable and unwilling to take responsibility for themselves (Furedi 2004). The government has had its own ideas about counselling and the role the talking therapies can perform (Department of Health 2007, 2008).

Counsellors themselves can find it difficult to say what counselling is, finding it easier to describe what counsellors do, the process and the hoped for outcomes. Some steer away from intended outcomes fearing this may seem that we will be directing clients to outcomes we see as hoped for and thus denying them autonomy.

Below are some of the things I have said in answer to the question 'What is counselling?'

> 'I help people work through their issues, difficulties.' This sounds very easy and simple.
> 'I listen to people and let them know what I have heard and understood from what they tell me.' This sounds easy, and if I add 'what they haven't said' it can sound scary too.
> 'I accept the person and don't judge their behaviour, but try to build a trusting relationship so the client can be open with me.' This sounds a bit superior and research tell us that clients choose not to tell us everything.

My honest answer to the question 'What is counselling?' is that counselling is hard work.

THE DEVELOPMENT OF COUNSELLING IN THE UNITED KINGDOM

Counselling is a social phenomenon of the latter part of the twentieth century, arising from the social, cultural and economic changes that began in the nineteenth century. These changes led to a reduction in the place of organised religion in the everyday life of many people. As the expectation and patterns of life changed, it became the norm for women to work rather than stay at home. The support networks of family and neighbours weakened as families broke apart and people moved away from the family home for work. People began to employ 'professionals' to do tasks they would have previously done themselves, for example painting and decorating, car maintenance and help with emotional difficulties. The result was a society in which people had more freedom and choice than earlier generations but the traditional sources of support, such as the extended family, the church and jobs for life had disappeared for many. The Welfare state and the National Health Service introduced after the Second World War came to provide an alternative to the support networks lost (Perkin 2002).

In order to understand the difficulty in the definition of counselling it is necessary to understand the origins and development of counselling in the United Kingdom. Many people equate the origins of counselling in the United Kingdom with the arrival of Carl Rogers' client-centred therapy in the late 1950s and 1960s. In fact, counselling had had a long and varied existence since the late nineteenth century and early twentieth century under other names.

Trying to identify the roots of counselling is similar to finding the source of the Nile. There are competing claims. What follows is a very short summary of the sources.

Counselling in the United Kingdom has deep historical roots originating in the various forms of help offered to the poor, both deserving and undeserving. This help came from the volunteers of the Charity Organisation Society (COS) and Police Court Missionaries. The court missionaries and Temperance officers were attached to police courts to help people found guilty of drunkenness. These workers were often linked to and employed by established churches in the early years. The COS volunteers, who were mainly middle-class women, worked with poor families and by the end of the nineteenth century were using what would be recognised today as a case work approach. These two groups developed into social workers and probation officers, with formal training for both introduced as early as 1903.

A second tributary arose from the spread of psychoanalytic ideas to treat soldiers suffering from shellshock after the First World War and the influence of the ideas of the Eugenics movement. These were put into practice in Child Guidance Clinics where by the 1930s psychiatric social workers were delivering psychodynamic therapy to clients. There was an increase in marriage breakdown and sexual violence after demobilisation of troops from the Second World War, leading to government anxiety about a potential threat to social cohesion (Hennessy 2007). This led to government funding for Marriage Guidance organisations, which were being overwhelmed by the demand for help. In order to have some confidence in the quality of the support on offer a Council was established to oversee training for the volunteer marriage guidance counsellors (Herbert and Jarvis 1970).

The introduction of the National Health Service and the Welfare state brought about a major change in the expansion of support services available to everyone, not just the poor. Social workers, psychiatric social workers, probation officers and clinical psychologists became state employed professionals. Others remained within the pastoral and charitable sectors and the Marriage Guidance Councils. In the immediate post-war period, most of these activities were not called 'counselling'. The term counselling came into use gradually after 1945 in the United Kingdom, especially in the Marriage Guidance Councils. Its use became more common with the arrival of Rogers' client-centred counselling.

From the 1960s onwards counselling expanded in the United Kingdom. As a result of the Newsome Report in 1963 and lobbying by the National Association for Mental Health (later to become MIND) postgraduate courses were set up in universities to train school counsellors. This was paralleled by the expansion of Marriage Guidance Councils and in the same period several religious based organisations were established and began to offer training, for example the Westminster Pastoral Foundation (WPF) and the Clinical Theology Association (CTA).

By the late 1960s this uncontrolled expansion of counselling was causing concern, as there were no common training standards or any definition of counselling. Government and charitable funding was provided to set up a Standing Conference for the Advancement of Counselling (SCAC). The organisations joining SCAC shows the breadth and range of counselling; it included universities, colleges, schools, professional organisations, psychoanalytic organisations, the medical colleges, government departments, the churches, Trade Unions, any and every organisation with an interest in counselling. In 1977 SCAC became the British Association for Counselling (BAC).

The wide range of interest groups in SCAC helps to explain why counselling often has a context-derived adjective attached to it, such as *school* counsellor, *marriage guidance* counsellor. It also helps to understand how counselling came to be used indiscriminately as an umbrella term to encompass a wide set of activities, many of which would not be seen as counselling today.

In the 1980s the government set up the National Council for Vocational Qualifications (NCVQ) and introduced a national framework for vocational qualifications (NVQs) to be delivered in the vocational sector, that is schools and Further Education colleges, not universities (see Chapter 5). 'Vocational', in this context, did not mean 'a calling' such as people feel who are drawn to entering a religious order, but vocational in the sense of skills-based, in contrast to academic- or thinking- and writing-based (see Chapter 2). The field of helping activities – counselling, befriending, counselling skills, advice, guidance and mediation – came together, and the first step was a project to differentiate between these activities (Russell, Dexter et al. 1992).

Counselling was defined in the Differentiation Project as,

> an activity entered into by a person seeking help, it offers the opportunity to identify things for the client themselves that are troubling or perplexing. It is clearly and explicitly contracted, and the boundaries of the relationship identified. The activity itself is designed to help self-exploration and understanding. The process should help to identify thoughts, emotions and behaviours that, once accessed, may offer the client the opportunity for a greater sense of personal resources and self determined change. (Russell, Dexter et al. 1992: 6)

In contrast, Counselling Skills were defined as,

> high level communication, interpersonal and social skills used intentionally in a manner consistent with the goals and values of counselling ethics. The principled use of these skills facilitates the client's purpose and enhances personal understanding of themselves and/or situations. As a direct result of using counselling skills the professional role of the user will be enhanced. (Russell, Dexter et al. 1992: 7)

Befriending was defined as being informal and opposed to professionalisation. Befriending has friends not clients: 'It seeks to share the problem or issue rather than manage or solve it' (Russell, Dexter et al. 1992: 5).

In contrast the working definition of guidance, while including the development of client self-awareness, stressed other aspects of the role, including 'To enable the client to be aware of and have access to accurate appropriate information on available opportunities in order to make informed choices' (Russell, Dexter et al. 1992: 7).

The Differentiation Project established counselling as a distinct activity with a set of competences that were developed into National Vocational Qualifications for counselling. These sit in a National Qualifications Framework to be delivered in the Further Education sector. Previously, counsellor training had been postgraduate courses delivered by universities or the qualifications of private training organisations such as Relate and WPF. In the 1990s the introduction of NVQs and other related qualifications led to an increase in the number and range of counselling qualifications, which were widely available in local Further Education Colleges. Many of these courses were and remain qualifications in counselling skills at Levels 2 and 3 on the Qualification and Credit Framework (QCF) (the Scottish Credit and Qualifications Framework (SCQF) in Scotland); others are professional training courses (see Chapter 3 on Training). When the output of all the training courses that aim to produce qualified counsellors and psychotherapists are added together, about 5,000 new counsellors and psychotherapists enter the field each year.

There was, however, a downside to this: the introduction of vocational qualifications in counselling contributed to a belief that counselling had no theoretical base, but was a set of skills to be acquired. This has persisted in a view that what a counsellor does depends on the setting of the work, not on any theoretical concepts and training. The increase in both demand and provision of counselling stimulated critical comment and observations on the nature and purpose of counselling and its function in society. For some, counselling in a social context, is 'a liberatory movement, committed to wresting power and authority from those who have assumed positions of authority in relation to ordinary peoples' everyday lives' (Bondi 2004). The goal of counselling is to facilitate the client's empowerment so that he/she can change their situation. This view sits alongside the view that counselling originally was 'an avowedly lay practice, constituted as something wholly different from a profession, and taking particular care to avoid making practitioners experts' (Bondi 2004: 320–1). There are strongly held views that the counselling relationship should be of equals, without hierarchy or expertise, embedded in everyday work (McLeod 2009). Professionalisation is anathema to counsellors who hold these beliefs; it represents the abandonment of the anti-authoritarian principles from which counselling sprang. Some voluntary counsellors oppose payment believing something would be lost if it was not voluntary: 'Volunteers do it for no other reason than the love of it, the desire for that relational contact' (Bondi 2004: 329). This view sees counselling as a process of mutual aid between peers, where one person is in distress or facing difficulties.

Allied with this view of counselling as a social movement is the opposition to the imposition of a medical model on counselling, with the idea of illness rather than *dis*-ease, diagnosis and treatment of symptoms with manuals for the treatment of each condition, approved centrally. This strongly held view believes in seeing the client as a whole rather than a presentation of symptoms, and within his/her social and cultural setting rather than as an individual in isolation.

Other views look at counselling in terms of its function in culture and society. Two of these views are presented here. The first sees counselling as a negative force in society, and the second sees it as an inadvertent agent of the state whose function is to support social stability.

Counselling, together with the other psychological therapies, psychiatry, psychology, and psychotherapy are accused of 'manufacturing victims' and creating a self-perpetuating business (Dineen 1999), setting themselves up as authorities in happiness and health (Evans 1999). The psychological therapies are seen as responsible for weakening the moral fibre of the population, by turning ordinary life events into problems that need expert psychological help to deal with, for example: 'A change in individual circumstance is often elevated into a problem that requires professional support'(Furedi 2004: 108). As traditional social support networks become less available, and people have lower expectation of their existing relationships, individuals are encouraged to use therapists as an alternative rather than dealing with the issues themselves. Thus 'therapeutic culture helps foster the perception of the self – as uniquely vulnerable and weak' (Furedi 2004: 105). In this argument the aim of counselling to empower the client towards understanding and autonomy is negated by the sense of helplessness created by this 'therapy culture'. The medicalisation of unhappiness and distress by the kind of diagnoses in the Diagnostic and Statistical Manual of Mental Disorders (DSM) means that individuals are not only unhappy and not coping, they are also diagnosed as sick. Commentators like Dineen (1999) and Furedi (2004) see the therapies as a self-serving business, with a vested interest in keeping clients helpless and dependent.

Another view of the therapies arises from the growth in emphasis on the individual in society and the use made of this by government. In other words, this is the direct opposite of the views that counselling is a subversive activity. There are two main strands to this proposition. When the subjective experience of the individual becomes of primary importance, that internal individual focus takes away attention from larger issues. People see problems as personal and their responsibility to resolve, rather than as the result of government policies (Rose 1985, 1990; Foucault 1991). This acts to stifle dissent, as dissatisfied individuals are not politically active but engrossed in their own counselling. The social and cultural value of giving so much attention to the private self is validated by a culture that encourages and applauds the celebrity private/ public self revelations.

The perspective of government on counselling and the other psychological therapies is that such psychological interventions may be useful if they can increase the wellbeing and functioning of the public. Government works to bring individual hopes, desires and fulfilment into line with its political goals and by so doing avoids any dissent. Counselling plays a role in maintaining this social stability by enabling the individual to regulate him/her self to fit in with the moral values and political principles of the day.

This may be difficult to swallow, but for evidence look at the changing goal of the Marriage Guidance Council/Relate – even the name shows how it changed from a goal of preserving marriages to working with relationships. In the recession of the 1970s the government invested in counselling for the unemployed and young people. The Improving Access to Psychological Therapies (IAPT) project 2008–12 can be interpreted in this way as a project to reduce the benefits bill through the delivery of certain types of therapy (Layard 2006; IAPT 2012). It was argued that the talking therapies, Cognitive Behavioural Therapy in particular, could be used to increase productivity and reduce the sickness benefits bill by keeping people in work or enabling them to return to work. In this view therapy 'is a sedative cynically administered to stifle dissidence and unrest … In short, therapy has become the opiate of the people' (Morrison 2003).

THE DEBATE ON THE DIFFERENCE BETWEEN COUNSELLING AND PSYCHOTHERAPY

There is an apocryphal story that a leading academic in the field when asked 'What is the difference between counselling and psychotherapy?' replied 'About £50 an hour'.

The issue of the difference or not between counselling and psychotherapy is one that divides counsellors and psychotherapists and the psychological therapy organisations. It is both caused by and one of the causes of the lack of a definition for counselling. Below are definitions of counselling and psychotherapy taken from a well respected book – *What Works for Whom?* (Roth and Fonagy 2005).

Counselling is:

> a term used to denote a varied set of techniques used to address a wide range of problems … Counselling is not a unitary theory or framework but tends to be defined by the setting in which it takes place … The focus is usually on current problems facing the individual, and the approach taken is frequently pragmatic ... it has also specialised to focus on particular clinical settings (such as primary care) or problems (such as bereavement). (Roth and Fonagy 2005: 13)

Psychotherapy is defined as distinguished by the following characteristics: 'the presence of a therapist–patient relationship; the interpersonal context of the psychotherapies and the implied notion of training and professionalism, the sense that therapies are conducted according to a model that guides the therapist's actions' (Strupp 1978: 3, quoted in Roth and Fonagy 2005: 5).

These definitions present counselling as lacking in theory, restricted in practice, with no mention of relationship or ethics. What is described as psychotherapy could equally well be applied to counselling. For example, other books in this series of Short Introductions present differing views: psychoanalysis lays claim to spawning counselling and psychotherapy (Milton, Polmear et al. 2011); psychotherapy claims differences in an overlapping field and acknowledges the confusion and lack of clear definition

(Lister-Ford 2007); and finally counselling psychology allies itself closely to counselling and psychotherapy to establish its distinctive nature within psychology (Orlans and Van Scoyoc 2009).

Attempts have been made to distinguish between counselling and psychotherapy but none have been wholly successful and there is no agreement on this issue. One distinction suggests that psychotherapists work with mental disorders and do longer-term, deeper work than counsellors. Another distinction is the identification of counsellors by the context of the work. Psychotherapists seem more likely than counsellors to work in private practice and less likely to be in paid employment, but this says nothing about the nature of that work (Aldridge and Pollard 2005). In the workplace, especially in education and the NHS, people with psychotherapy qualifications will be employed as counsellors. The IAPT programme dealt with the problem by employing High Intensity Therapists, who are mainly clinical psychologists qualified in Cognitive Behavioural Therapy (CBT).

One of the distinctions made has been to see counselling as vocational, that is skills based, with little theoretical or research base and psychotherapy as more academic and a science. Another distinction has linked psychotherapy to mental illness and a medical model of patients and treatment, as opposed to counselling's clients and process. This distinction comes directly from the historical origins of counselling and psychotherapy. There have been attempts to link counselling with wellbeing rather than mental illness as some counsellors dislike the use of a medical model of diagnosis and treatment for what they see as 'problems of living'.

Counsellors understand clients from a wider perspective than diagnosis of illness and treatment; they see and work with a whole person. For example, with a bereaved client a counsellor might wonder about how this loss fits with both the current life and social world of the client and previous losses, the impact on the sense of identity and value of the client and facilitate the need to grieve. Other professional groups might wish to assess symptoms of depression and ways to deal with these. The client might experience both as equally helpful and supportive. In some cases the difference may rest in semantics, how the client or patient describes the issue that has brought them for help.

As there is no legal restriction on the use of the titles counsellor and psychotherapist, practitioners are free to describe themselves as they choose. It seems that most stay with the title of their first training, although some describe themselves as psychotherapists for private practice and are also employed as counsellors (Aldridge and Pollard 2005).

Perhaps the clearest summary of the situation is set out below, but it must be borne in mind that this is made by the BACP which sees no difference between counselling and psychotherapy:

Despite numerous attempts by organisations and individuals to distinguish between the knowledge base, skills, responsibilities and activities associated with counselling and psychotherapy, there is no reliable evidence that indicates any significant difference. It is clear that the descriptive title given to professional psychological therapists depends largely on the core theoretical model to which they adhere, the setting in which they practise, and to some extent on the training they have received. Both terms are used to describe the explicitly contracted therapeutic process through which personal concerns are described, explored and processed. The term counselling has its origins in the word counsel, meaning 'to advise', but in contemporary professional practice advice is not part of normal practice.

Counselling and psychotherapy are umbrella terms that cover a range of talking therapies. They are delivered by trained practitioners who work with people over the short or long term to help them bring about effective change and enhance their wellbeing. Counselling and psychotherapy can be hugely beneficial for many people in a wide variety of situations including helping people to cope with depression and anxiety, bereavement, relationship difficulties, sexual and racial issues, child abuse and educational dilemmas, as well as personal problem solving. Therapy offers people a safe, confidential place to talk about life issues and problems that may be confusing, painful or uncomfortable. (see www.bacp.co.uk/admin/structure/files/pdf/7461_gtt_briefing.pdf)

The distinction seemed of relatively little importance until the 2007 Act, Trust Assurance and Safety, which stated the intention to statutorily regulate psychology, counselling and psychotherapy. The growing popularity and demand for counselling led to the inclusion of counselling in the New Labour government's list of psychological professions to be subject to the statutory regulation in the Health Professions Council (HPC, now the Health and Care Professions Council). The inclusion of counselling alongside psychology and psychotherapy in the 2007 Act, Trust Assurance and Safety, was a form of recognition – a recognition that counselling presented enough risk to the public to be subject to statutory control. For many this was seen as a positive form of recognition and status.

Statutory regulation is based on the legal protection of title, meaning that someone could only call themselves a counsellor if they had done the HPC's approved training and were on the HPC's register for that title. The purpose of statutory regulation was public protection by imposing standards for entry to the profession and a complaints procedure by which someone could be removed from the register and therefore prevented from practising. Psychologists were regulated first in the Health Professions Council with nine separate titles, including clinical and counselling psychologist. The HPC established a Professional Liaison Group to set the standards for the titles of counsellor and psychotherapist. This process was dominated by attempts to establish and codify the difference. One of the suggested differences proposed that counsellors worked on wellbeing and psychotherapists worked on mental health issues. It was also suggested that counsellors required a lower level of training than psychotherapists. This proposed differentiation drew protests from working counsellors who worked with mental health issues and also those who held postgraduate degrees. There were similar protests from psychotherapists who believed that standards would be lowered if counsellors with postgraduate qualifications were given similar status to psychotherapists. In 2010 the change of government led to a change of policy towards the regulation and quality control of professionals. The policy of statutory regulation was replaced by a quality assurance scheme for voluntary registers for unregulated health and social care occupational groups, administered by the Professional Standards Authority for Health and Social Care. This is covered in more detail in Chapter 8.

THE DEVELOPMENT OF THE TALKING THERAPIES

Historically it is possible to see four separate strands in the development of the talking therapies – the scientific strand that is represented by clinical psychology with an emphasis on scientific research, psychoanalysis with its focus on talking as a way to address problems arising from the individual psyche, counselling as a social support movement and humanistic counselling as an alternative to the dominance of psychoanalysis. Psychotherapy appears in each of these, but first emerged in psychoanalysis where the term was used for non-medical or lay analysts.

The first talking therapists were the medical psychoanalysts, for example Freud. The title 'counsellor' came into use after the end of the Second World War, first in the voluntary sector and later in schools and colleges. Clinical psychologists emerged as part of the National Health Service in 1948, but psychologists were relatively late to recognise the growth of counselling, only establishing the Counselling Psychology Division in the British Psychological Society in 1995. The term psychotherapist has been in existence since the early twentieth century, at the start denoting lay analysts. The term as it is understood today usually refers to members of the organisations that formed the Standing Conference for the Advancement of Psychotherapy (1989), now known as the United Kingdom Council for Psychotherapy.

Today, talking therapists are made up of counsellors, psychoanalysts, psychiatrists, clinical and counselling psychologists, and psychotherapists.

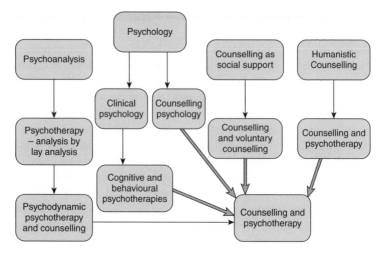

Figure 1.1 *The development of the talking therapies*

There are differences in these groups that must be acknowledged; psychiatrists and psychologists require specific first degrees in the subject area before moving into postgraduate training as psychological therapists. These two groups therefore hold the highest level of academic qualifications. By contrast, psychoanalysts may take as many, if not more years in training, but usually without formal academic qualifications. Psychotherapists tend to train with private training schools, like the psychoanalysts, but many psychotherapy trainings have gained validation as postgraduate qualifications. Counsellors can train at any level from 4 to doctorate.

Figure 1.1 summarises the development of the talking therapies.

COUNSELLING AS A PROFESSION

Another question arises when trying to define counselling: 'Is counselling a profession?' Or, put another way, 'Are counsellors professionals?' Counselling is seen by some people as representing a group of people, often volunteers, with little training, who listen to people sympathetically and try to help or who are 'embedded counsellors' (McLeod 2009) using counselling within another role. This first group would eschew professional status as having negative connotations. A research project with voluntary counsellors in Scotland found that they believed professional status would damage the therapeutic work with clients by making the counsellor seem superior, rather than equal (Bondi 2004). There is also a history of counselling being seen as an activity and set of values that should be practised and embraced by wide sections of society (Halmos 1967; McLeod 2009). Others fear that creativity and freedom would be constrained by becoming a profession (House and Totton 1997). There are many thousands of counsellors for whom counselling is their main occupation and how they define themselves. These counsellors welcome the status of a professional, seeing it as recognition of the training, supervision and ethical work they undertake.

This group's claim to professional status can be undermined by a view that counsellors are very much part-time volunteers with little training and therefore limited competence. Added to this is a view that counselling is 'vocational' rather than 'professional' as counsellors are taught to use 'skills' just like builders and car mechanics. Professionals on the other hand have academic and intellectual training and work with the 'mind not the 'hands.' This is clearly nonsense when looking at what a counsellor does in a session with a client. Research with clients shows that the expectation is that counsellors are trained and qualified professionals (Forsythe and Corfino 2008).

The BACP, which is the largest professional association for counsellors and psychotherapists in the UK, is in no doubt that counselling is a profession. Laurie Clarke, the Chief Executive Officer, recently wrote about the BACP's Register gaining accreditation from the Professional Standards Authority:

> This accreditation is great news for counsellors, psychotherapists and their clients. By recognising the important role the profession plays in the country's health and emotional wellbeing, it will give our members the status within the health and social care sector that they deserve. (www.bacp.co.uk/media)

CONCLUSION

While it may not be possible to create a short, clear definition for counselling or even for the psychological therapies, one thing is known about therapy: 'that most people who have had therapy feel that is has benefited them in some way' (Evans 1999).

Counselling can be defined by its purpose, to enable the client to gain in confidence and ability to deal with future problems on their own. Counselling aims to remove the stigma from seeking help for distress. Paul Halmos, in the 1960s, hoped that the values and attitudes of counselling would pervade society, but acknowledged as he wrote that he was an optimist (Halmos 1964, 1967). But research since has found that hope is an important aspect of successful counselling. When the counsellor believes that what they offer can help, this can have a powerful positive impact on the client. It is almost as if such belief and hope can be infectious.

Not everyone sees the growth of counselling and the talking therapies as positive. Some see counselling's encouragement of self-knowledge and self-reflection as a form of 'self-surveillance' that can encourage social conformity and compliance (Rose 1990). Another view claims that the growth of psychological help offered by counselling has had at least two negative outcomes. The first is the emphasis on the importance of the individual rather than the family or wider community; thus encouraging selfishness rather than generosity or altruism. The second is that the therapies encourage clients into dependent relationships and a belief that they are 'ill' rather than distressed and unhappy (Furedi 2004). This latter argument appears to misunderstand the purpose of counselling to enable the client to deal with the issues and difficulties enough to be able to get back to functioning independently.

The disputes and struggles for superiority and status within the psychological therapies have hampered the development of a clear definition of counselling. For many people within the talking therapies, counselling is seen as having lower status in relation to the other professional groups, so definitions that do not reflect this do not gain acceptance within the field. Ironically some of these people are employed as counsellors, because the public demand is for counselling.

The lack of a short, simple, well-understood definition of counselling can be both an advantage and a disadvantage. When working with the civil servants responsible for the IAPT programme, I was asked more than once, what is counselling? They had evidence from the outcome statistics that 'counselling' was getting good outcomes and wanted to increase the amount on offer. The problem was that the category was 'counselling' without any further detail, as opposed to 'cognitive behavioural therapy'. The outcome was the commissioning of three additional forms of counselling – humanistic counselling, dynamic interpersonal therapy and behavioural couples therapy.

The author is not going to attempt a definition of counselling. This chapter should have made it clear that this would be thankless and unsuccessful. What happens in counselling is that someone puts aside their own concerns and gives attention to another person in a formal agreed way, where the goal is to help the other person gain a better understanding of what is troubling them and maybe make some changes. This is done in a formal contracted relationship in which the counsellor works ethically within his/her competence. Counselling has authority; this authority comes from 'its ability to give meaning to experience in a world strongly wedded to a therapeutic ethos' (Furedi 2004: 10).

Activity

Counselling is seen as:

1 Having no theoretical foundation.
2 Being the application of skills to a problem.
3 Being an everyday activity that anyone who wants to can do.
4 Being voluntary rather than professional or paid.

How do you respond to each of these statements?
Does your experience and knowledge fit with any of these statements?

Activity

How would you define counselling?
Find a range of definitions of counselling using internet search engines, dictionaries, counselling and psychotherapy organisations, government website.
Compare these to the definitions in this chapter and your own definition. What are the common elements?
What is missing from some of them?

REFERENCES

Aldridge, S. and J. Pollard (2005). *Interim Report on the Mapping of Counselling and Psychotherapy*. London, Department of Health.

Bondi, L. (2004). 'A double-edged sword? The professionalisation of counselling in the United Kingdom', *Health & Place* **10**(4): 319–28.

Catty, J. (2010). *Making Sense of Counselling*. London, Mind.

Department of Health (2007). *Trust, Assurance and Safety – The Regulation of Health Professionals in the 21st Century*. London, Department of Health.

Department of Health (2008). *Improving Access to Psychological Therapies (IAPT) Commissioning Toolkit*. London, Department of Health.

Dineen, T. (1999). *Manufacturing Victims: What the Psychology Industry is Doing to People*, London, Constable.

ENTO (2008). *Labour Market Intelligence Survey*. Employment National Training Organisation (ENTO)

Evans, D. (1999). 'A sickness called therapy. Review of *Manufacturing Victims. What the Psychology Industry is Doing to People* by Tana Dineen', *Guardian* 28 August 1999.

Forsythe, N. and Corfino, S. (2008). *Counsellors, Psychotherapists and User. How to become More Customer-centric.* London: commissioned by BACP.

Foucault, M. (1991). 'Governmentality'. In G. Burchell, C. Gordon and P. Miller (Eds), *The Foucault Effect Studies in Governmentality.* Chicago, University of Chicago Press: 87–104.

Furedi, F. (2004). *Therapy Culture.* London, Routledge.

Halmos, P. (1964). *The Faith of the Counsellors.* Edinburgh: Constable.

Halmos, P. (1967). 'The personal service society', *British Journal of Sociology* **18**: 13–28.

Hennessy, P. (2007). *Having It So Good. Britain in the Fifties.* London, Penguin.

Herbert, W. L. and F. V. Jarvis (1970). *Marriage Counselling in the Community.* Oxford, Pergamon Press.

House, R. and N. Totton (Eds) (1997). *Implausible Professions. Arguments for Pluralism and Autonomy in Psychotherapy and Counselling.* Llangoarron, PCCS Books.

IAPT (2012). *IAPT 3 Year Report. The first million patients.* London: Department of Health.

Layard, R. (2006). *The Depression Report. A new deal for depression and anxiety disorders.* London, The Centre for Economic Performance, London School of Economics.

Lister-Ford, C. (Ed.) (2007). *A Short Introduction to Psychotherapy. Short Introduction to the Therapy Professions.* London, Sage.

McLeod, J. (2009). *An Introduction to Counselling.* Maidenhead, Open University Press.

Mental Health Foundation, Mind., et al. (2006). *We Need to Talk. The case for psychological therapy on the NHS.* London: Mental Health Foundation.

Milton, J., C. Polmear, et al. (2011). *A Short Introduction to Psychoanalysis.* London, Sage.

Morrison, B. (2003). 'Cultivating vulnerability in an uncertain age. Review of *Therapy Culture* by Frank Furedi', *Guardian* 20 December 2003: 10.

Orlans, V. and S. Van Scoyoc (2009). *A Short Introduction to Counselling Psychology.* London, Sage.

Perkin, H. (2002). *The Rise of Professional Society.* London, Routledge.

Rose, N. (1985). *Psychological Complex, Psychology, Politics and Society in England 1869–1939.* London, Routledge and Keegan Paul.

Rose, N. (1990). *Governing the Soul, the Shaping of the Private Self.* London, Routledge Keegan Paul.

Roth, A. and P. Fonagy (2005). *What Works for Whom? A Critical Review of Psychotherapy Research.* New York, Guildford Press.

Russell, J., G. Dexter, et al. (1992). *Differentiation between Advice, Guidance, Befriending, Counselling skills and Counsellling.* Welwyn, The Advice, Guidance and Counselling Lead Body: 8.

Standing Conference for the Advancement of Counselling (1978). *What is Counselling?* London, SCAC.

2 COUNSELLING SKILLS AND THEIR APPLICATION IN WIDER SETTINGS

INTRODUCTION

This chapter looks at the differences between counselling skills and counselling and provides a definition of counselling skills. The differences were outlined in Chapter 1 and are further developed in this chapter. In everyday life, most of us, at times, use the skills that are collectively described as 'counselling skills'. We may do this when we listen to a friend or try to support a partner or child. Some of us also use these skills at work. Some people use counselling skills to enhance a professional role, for example a nurse or teacher: for others, such as befrienders, counselling skills are the heart of that role. Although the focus of this chapter is on the difference, it needs to be understood that counsellors use counselling skills all the time in their work and a vast range of other people use the same skills in other roles and contexts.

Many counsellors start by taking a counselling skills course and move on to professional training. Many more people take these courses and integrate the knowledge skills and values into their work. This chapter outlines the various settings in which counselling skills are used and the consequences of these different settings. It considers some of the ethical and personal challenges that can face the counselling skills user. The range and nature of training in counselling skills is outlined together with a brief description of the skills.

Some readers will have already undertaken counselling skills training courses, others will be considering this. There are many reasons for undertaking a counselling skills course. You may have noticed for example that people tend to tell you about their problems and want to be more confident that you are doing good not harm in how you respond. You may want to find out what helping people in this way involves, and whether you can do it. Curiosity about oneself can also be a motive. It can be something as ordinary as that the only course at your local college on your free evening is the one on counselling skills. Some people have decided to train as a counsellor and a counselling skills course is the first stage of that training. Counselling skills courses are valuable in their own right.

A physiotherapist working in the NHS took a counselling skills course, because he had become aware that treating the physical problem on its own didn't seem enough. He said, 'Most physio patients don't improve because they don't follow the programme. I wanted to know if there was a way to change this.' He wanted to be able to understand and respond to the whole person as this would be more effective in terms of the patient's recovery. If he could understand the patient better, encourage the patient to talk to him, he would be better able to work out treatment programmes that the patient would actually do.

The manager of a team delivering training and events wanted to learn more about what made people become angry and why he found it difficult to respond to angry callers in an assertive way. Two other students on the course had decided that they wanted to make a career change and become counsellors.

INTERPERSONAL SKILLS OR COUNSELLING SKILLS?
IS THERE A DIFFERENCE?

Counselling skills derive from communication skills, social skills, inter-personal skills; it is the context and intention that makes them counselling skills. Counselling skills enable us to help other people by listening to them and communicating in ways that help the other person to talk about what concerns them, and by doing this to feel better or be able to see things more clearly. This way of communicating differs from ordinary conversation as the focus is on the other person.

One might think that if the context is 'right' the interpersonal and com-munication skills used in that context will always be counselling skills. For example, one would expect health care professionals to use counselling skills. However, if the task of the physiotherapist is to teach the patient how to use a pair of crutches so that she can be discharged from hospital, the technical instructions are the focus of that interaction, not how the patient feels about being discharged. Not all health professionals use counselling skills in all their interactions.

The difference between counselling skills and interpersonal or com-munication skills is the purpose for which they are used. The skills are counselling skills when they are used in the best interests of the recipient not in the interest of the user. This however, is a bit fuzzy – a car salesman could argue that he was using the skills in the recipient's best interests to find him/her the car that best suited, regardless of any bonus or commis-sion. But if counselling skills are used to direct or gain advantage from a client then the skills no longer have the philosophical underpinning and ethical framework of counselling and are communications skills.

One way to identify the difference is very practical – who is doing the talking? Tim Bond (2010) suggests that this makes clear when counselling skills are being employed. From Table 2.1 it is clear that when using counselling skills, the user aims to speak for less time, and to make sure what he/she does say communicates that the recipient has been heard and understood. This differs from ordinary conversation as the focus is on the other person.

Table 2.1   *Patterns of communication flow*

Style of communication	Pattern of flow of communication	Speaking ratio
Imparting expertise	Interactor to recipient	80:20
Ordinary conversation	Interactor to recipient	50:50
Using counselling skills	Interactor to recipient	20:80

Source: Bond (2010)

Counselling skills are linked to the objectives of the person using them. For example a police officer may be surprised and unsure why an elderly widow whose house has been burgled is adamant that she does not want any information about or help from the Victim Support Service. The officer could have accepted this, but decided to use counselling skills to try to find out a bit more about the reason. He found out that the victim feared that she had not had the window locks on and that the burglary was her fault. He was able to reassure her that it had been a forced entry through a locked window.

Years ago, I was a couple of months into my training as a counsellor. One evening I was Christmas shopping with my husband. I noticed the salesman just taking the weight off one foot. I said something like, 'Your feet must ache on long days like this,' and we got into a conversation about his job. I was thrilled to find that the skills worked in everyday life and how good I felt after the interaction. My soon-to-be ex-husband on the other hand thought we had both wasted his time. In this interaction neither I nor the salesperson were consciously or deliberately entering into a counselling skills interaction. I was trying out some skills I had recently learnt. He was pleased to have someone to talk to. One thing users of counselling skills quickly learn, as I did, is their power, and the good feelings generated in both people by the interaction. I cannot place responsibility for my subsequent career in counselling on that salesman, but I do wonder if the interaction had been different, what my future might have been. As it was, I was hooked – I could be interested in people without being accused of being nosy and intrusive; I could be nice to people and they would respond.

THE DIFFERENCES BETWEEN COUNSELLING AND COUNSELLING SKILLS

Work role

Counselling is delivered by someone whose role/occupation is that of a counsellor. Many counsellors work in structured settings with clients who have chosen to come to a professional for help. Many counselling skills users use the skills to enhance their main occupational role (nurse, teacher), but not to change that role to one of counsellor.

Purpose

Counselling has a theoretical framework, ethical boundaries and a purposeful intent that goes beyond the purpose of enhancing a professional role, which is often the main aim of the use of counselling skills. Counselling skills is the use of communication and social skills in a way consistent with the values, goals and communications patterns of counselling. When used intentionally, counselling skills reflect the values of counselling, to assist the self-expressions and autonomy of the helpee. Counselling skills are not a role in themselves. They are used to enhance the performance of other roles including befriending, advising, giving guidance and counselling and to enhance the performance of other occupational relationships, such as nurse–patient, teacher–student, policeman–citizen.

If a social worker uses these skills to better communicate with a client and get a better understanding of the issues, these are counselling skills. If used to direct or gain advantage from a client then the skills lose the philosophical underpinning and ethical frame and are just a use of communications skills.

Relationships and expectations

Both counselling skills user and the recipient/helpee will have expectations of the relationship, or often more accurately, relationships. There are the obvious differences between counsellors and counselling skills users in terms of the confidentiality, the boundaries and the contractual nature of the relationship. There are other differences. The recipient of counselling skills sees the practitioner as carrying out his/her primary role, which is not that of a counsellor. Therefore, the recipient will not regard him/herself as being a counselling client, but as whatever the recipient of the main role might be – patient, student, victim of a crime, a solicitor's client, etc. The user's main role may be enhanced by the use of counselling skills but the recipient responds to the primary role. Thus the lady who was burgled was talking to a police officer, not a counselling skills user or a counsellor.

Contracts

In counselling there will be an explicit contract and the client has made a conscious decision to enter counselling. The contract with a client will cover such things as where and when to meet; for how long in terms of session length, frequency and possibly duration of the counselling; the fees if any, policy on cancellations and emergency contact and the limits of confidentiality. This contract may be made by the agency, the counsellor or a combination of the two. It may also include issues such as what to expect in counselling, the theoretical approach used and how to make a complaint. In other words, there is no doubt in the mind of the recipient that he/she is entering a formal therapeutic counselling relationship with boundaries.

The recipient of counselling skills does not expect to enter into the sort of explicit contract as he/she would with a counsellor. Counselling skills users have a different relationship, in terms of the confidentiality, the boundaries and the contractual nature of the relationship. This may be an explicit contract with the user's other role, for example tutoring, befriending, supporting or mentoring.

Sometimes the context may give rise to forms of contract depending on the role of the counselling skills user, for example covering aspects of confidentiality. However, the interactions are often more informal or embedded within another role and indeed, the recipient may not be directly aware of the use of counselling skills at all, but will feel heard, respected and understood.

For example: a member of a staff network which supports employees who feel they have been subject to discrimination or bullying at work will have limits of confidentiality and actions which will be made clear when an employee approaches them. Anyone approaching a network member will expect to be listened to, treated with respect and to have an agreement about the confidentiality of what is discussed. This will not include an explicit contract for the use of counselling skills although these will be used in the interaction

THEORY

A counsellor will have trained in a particular theoretical approach and will be guided by this in work with clients. Counselling skills users will not have had such in-depth theoretical training. As a result a counselling skills user may not be so constrained in their responses, and at the same time will need to be aware of the limits of their competence.

Ethical requirements

Counselling skills users often have a different relationship, in terms of the ethical aspects of the relationship. For example, there is unlikely to be a contract for the specific use of counselling skills between the two parties. The problems presented by confidentiality and boundaries are considered in more detail later. A counsellor is bound by the ethics and standards of their training and profession, and accountable to the client and professional association. Whilst a counsellor is ethically bound to serve the best interests of the client, in some circumstances this can be a conflict of interest for a counselling skills user. The counselling skills user may be bound by the ethical codes of his/her core profession and may have to work out possible ethical conflicts of interest.

Limits of competence and referrals

Counsellors have undertaken substantial training and work within a specific theoretical model with a set of ethical values. Such training includes risk assessment and knowledge of mental health issues. (See QAA benchmarks for counselling and psychotherapy.) Counselling skills users recognise the limits of their competence with respect to counselling and need to know when and how to make appropriate referrals and to whom.

Supervision

Counsellors are required to have regular supervision of work with clients. There is no similar requirement for supervision for people using counselling skills. Some professions in which counselling skills are used do have supervision, but the focus of the supervision will be different.

Practical differences – setting and duration

Counsellors work within fixed time slots of sessions and numbers of sessions of counselling. Counselling skills users in some roles may have similar work patterns, for example, nurses running specialist clinics, sports coaches; but others do not – for example, Trade Union officials. Often they are called upon to use the skills with no warning and no knowledge of the possible length of the interaction. Counsellors work in dedicated rooms, providing a high level of privacy. Counselling skills users may find themselves in public places or open plan offices or wards, where privacy is limited.

Types of counselling skills users

People who use counselling skills consciously can be divided into two groups. The first group comprise people in the caring or helping professions such as teachers, health care workers, nurses, social workers, youth and community workers, and those working in the voluntary sectors, etc. (Further reading is given at the end of the chapter.) These professionals regularly come into contact with people who are distressed, both physically and emotionally, and it is the task of the professional to help them. The prime task is to perform the key role: a doctor's prime role is to elicit the symptoms from the patients in order to diagnose the illness and find a suitable remedy; the lecturer's primary role is to support students in their learning through teaching and assessment. Both may choose to use counselling skills to explore the emotional state of the patient or student, the family circumstances, the expectations and hopes. A physiotherapist working with a patient to restore mobility may choose to use counselling skills to explore the motivation to improve, and discover that the patient enjoys being looked after by his/her partner and so has little motivation to change. With another patient, she may explore the emotional impact of long-term disability and discover depths of emotional distress that lead to a referral to counselling.

A pastoral care worker describes the value of counselling skills when working with elderly house-bound parishioners: 'I know how to sit and listen and how important it is to have someone take an interest and really want to know. Usually it isn't about changing anything, more about me being there with them, understanding.'

The second group of people who use counselling skills are most accurately described as 'befrienders', for example the Samaritans and Age UK's befriending service. For these groups, counselling skills are at the heart of the work they do to provide support and listening to people who are isolated and finding life difficult.

The purpose of using counselling skills in all these roles is to support and respect the recipient and provide a space in which they can talk about issues. This may be a teacher talking through assignments with a pupil or a practice nurse talking about the management of diabetes, a youth worker talking to teenagers in a snooker hall. All these interactions will flow better and have better outcomes for both parties if counselling skills are skilfully employed by the professional in the best interests of the recipient. It may be frustrating for the practice nurse running the diabetes clinic to note that yet again a particular patient has not followed the diet and exercise routine. The use of non-judgemental listening and responding might help the nurse understand the patient's point of view, reveal the reason and enable the patient to consider how to address the issue, with the nurse's support.

This is not to say that in all interactions the focus should be on the use of counselling skills in the ways described above. In some circumstances, for example, it is more important that a pharmacist give clear instructions on medication than empathise with the recipient's illness.

DEFINITION AND DESCRIPTION OF COUNSELLING SKILLS

Definition

As we have noted with the technical communication, social and interpersonal skills, these skills need to be used with the addition of the values and attitudes of counselling. These attitudes and values of respect, acceptance and empathy are essential for the development of trust in the relationship. Counselling skills are the combination of attitude, values and skills used in the best interests of the recipient, aimed at helping that person better understand whatever issue is of concern to them. Privacy and confidentiality are not always essential for the use of counselling skills, although sometimes these are necessary.

BACP defines counselling skills as 'when there is an intentional use of inter-personal skills which reflects the values of counselling and the user's primary role is enhanced, without them taking on the role of counsellor and the recipient perceives the use as acting within their primary professional caring role, which is not that of being a counsellor.'

Description

The skills neatly divide into attention giving and responding skills. Attention giving skills involve listening carefully and giving full attention to the speaker, noticing the non-verbal communications between yourself and the recipient. Much depends on the tone of the words, posture and look of the person. All of these give indications of how the person is feeling. When giving attention, the aim is to receive the whole message from the other person, this includes the words said, the meaning given to those words and the emotions involved. In addition to the words said, we gather understanding from the tone used and non-verbal language such as facial expressions, how the person moves or sits. This is a two-way process and the other person will also be aware of your non-verbal communications. We seem to lack control over our non-verbal 'leakage' to each other and often respond to that more than to verbal communication.

It isn't safe to assume that the meaning of certain words and phrases to you is the same as it is to the other person. We all use figures of speech, particular phrases, metaphors; this makes it more difficult to understand what someone is really saying. In my family, the answer 'I'm nobbut mid-dling' to the question 'How are you?' can mean – 'I'm the same as usual, nothing much to complain about'. It can also mean 'I'm in a bad way and in need of some help.'

Responding skills have two aims. The first is to show that you have understood the other person accurately. Checking and clarifying your understanding helps build the relationship as it shows that the listener is genuinely concerned to get an accurate picture, this in turn builds empathy. This involves the use of paraphrases and summaries of what has been said, in such a way that the speaker feels understood but not interrupted in the flow of their communication. Feeding back to the person in a para-phrase or summary what you have understood can lead to clarification of what was previously vague and unformed to the recipient. Such para-phrasing and summarising also gives the recipient the opportunity to amend or correct both your and their understanding. The potential for multiple misunderstandings is neatly given in the well known sentence below, which has variously been attributed to Richard Nixon, Robert McClusky and Alan Greenspan among others:

'I know you think you understand what you thought I said, but I'm not sure you realise that what you heard is not what I meant.'

People do not of course paraphrase or summarise everything they have heard. Each of us will be selective and base that selection consciously on the other things picked up from the other person that might indicate an emphasis or importance to some elements over others. People will also unconsciously select some things above others. Figures 2.1 and 2.2 show the consequences of both good and poor attending and respond-ing skills.

The second aim is to assist the person to continue exploring the con-cern or issue. Paraphrasing and open questions can help the recipient focus more clearly on the issue or the options open to them. One set of skills are called 'miminal encouragers'. I have always thought this was a weighty phrase to give to such things as the 'Mms' and 'Ahs' and nods we use to keep conversation going. Sometimes responding skills also aim to help the recipient become aware of apparent contradictions, for example, between what they say and their behaviour. These are described as chal-lenging skills and must be used carefully only when the relationship is one of trust and understanding, or the recipient can feel under attack. One responding skill that may seem the opposite of responding is silence. Being comfortable with another person's silence when your purpose is to help them, is difficult to learn and accept. In these circumstances, it helps to go back to trusting in the other person and the fact that they are being silent with you.

In this interaction, the initial response was accurate and empathic. The second was inaccurate, but the respondent felt secure enough to correct the counselling skills user and the subsequent interaction showed a high level of attending and responding skills and empathy.

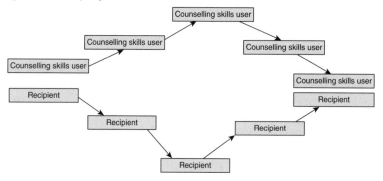

Figure 2.1   *Consequences of good attention giving and responding skills*

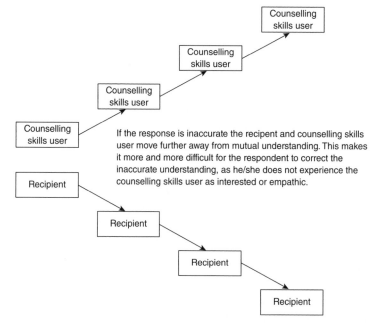

Figure 2.2   *Consequences of poor attention giving and responding skills*

In addition the counselling skills user must try to set aside personal views and opinions and be accepting of those expressed by the other person. He/she must also try to understand the feelings and experience of the other person and be accepting and non-judgemental. This can be very difficult when there seems to be an obvious solution, or the views being expressed are objectionable to the counselling skills user. Counsellors face the same problem.

So many things can get in the way of employing these skills. People can be anxious that they will get it wrong. So concerned to work out what the best paraphrase response will be they forget to listen and miss the thing that is really important to the other person. The chair might be uncomfortable, the sound proofing less than perfect. Our own value judgements can easily get in the way. All of these get in the way of the listening and responding of both counselling skills users and counsellors. It is important in the listening and responding to try to recognise the feelings and respond to these. If someone is telling you about a disappointing holiday with a new partner, an accurate summary of the holiday itinerary will not be the best use of counselling skills. A more helpful response would be focused on the disappointed expectations of the relationship and the possible options arising from that.

BOUNDARIES AND OTHER TRICKY ISSUES IN USING COUNSELLING SKILLS

Unintended consequences: existing relationships

One issue to consider is whether deliberately using counselling skills in relationships will change the nature of those relationships. In social settings I don't tell people I am a counsellor, I want to enjoy myself, not listen to other people's problems. If previously you have balanced interactions with friends, it is a good idea to monitor this to see if the balance has changed and if you are happy with this (see Table 2.1 on page 24). Good listeners can find it hard to be listened to when they need it. In addition, using counselling skills requires a high level of attention and concentration and receiving the distress and feelings is emotionally draining. It is ethical and sensible to ask yourself: 'Can I cope with what I might hear?' If there is an existing relationship, how might that be affected?

The counselling skills user can always steer the conversation away from areas he/she feels they cannot cope with. It is always possible to close down a subject, by choosing not to respond in ways that would encourage further exploration. Counselling skills users are not tied to a 50-minute counselling hour.

People who use counselling skills in other roles may lack the protection of the boundaries and structures a professional counsellor enjoys. The counselling skills user has to make on-the-spot decisions about whether to take the counselling skills approach with its focus on the best interests of the other person. Sometimes, this may be straightforward, such as a lack of time or suitable place to talk; it may be more complex and involve unintended and negative consequences for the counselling skills user.

Often the place and subject determines the nature of the interaction. For example, a lecturer may use communication skills in a disciplinary meeting with a student who has plagiarised an essay. The intention is to ensure the student understands the nature of the offence and the sanctions imposed. The same lecturer may have a meeting with a student whose grades have suddenly dropped, and the lecturer wants to help the student to understand the problem and consider the options available to address it. In this case the skills are counselling skills as the lecturer is concerned to understand the student and offer a safe supportive environment in which to explore the problem. Sometimes it will be right to offer suggestions, especially if you have this expertise in the primary role, as long as this is not an attempt to impose your solution. To withhold such information because you are in a counselling skills interaction may not be in the best interests of the recipient.

Unintended consequences

What if the lecturer dealing with the student guilty of plagiarism uses counselling skills to understand what led to the behaviour and as a result of what is revealed, imposes a lighter sanction? This could lead to accusations of favouritism, be challenged in terms of a breach of University policy on sanctions for plagiarism. It could easily result in a stream of students with hard luck stories expecting similar mitigation.

Positions of authority

A second important point in the interaction between the lecturer and the student is that the lecturer is in a position of authority. Managers may find that appraisals and performance reviews are more productive and positive when using counselling skills, but the manager is in the position of authority and needs to remember this. People using counselling skills as befrienders or buddies may self-disclose as a part of the development of the relationship; people who hold authority need to take more care and give thought to the possible consequences of self-disclosure to subordinate work colleagues.

Dual roles

Many users of counselling skills will already have a relationship with the person with whom they are using the skills, for example the nurse and the patient, the teacher and the pupil. Sometimes, there may be multiple roles. A middle manager could be a member of the Trade Union and the company's mentoring scheme, and in the same pub quiz team as the person seeking some support.

The recipient will see the counselling skills user in whatever role they are in when the interaction takes place and not as a counselling skills user per se. The use of the skills should be subtle and not a jarring change in the nature of the interaction. For example a supervisor who makes a sudden switch from a critical performance review about missed targets to an empathic listener about how that all feels, is not likely to engender trust in the recipient. Dual and multiple roles need to be managed, especially when they give rise to conflicts of interest (Gabriel 2005).

Conflicts of interest

The use of counselling skills must be in the best interests of the recipient; this does not mean that the user of counselling skills should ignore the possible consequences to themselves in their primary role. Conflicts of interest can arise between using counselling skills and the user's primary role. Take for example a home care worker who has a list of eleven elderly people to visit each morning. The fifth person in the list had an upsetting conversation with his niece the evening before; she had been trying to persuade him that it was time to go into residential care. He is clearly upset and wants to talk about it. The support worker may use her counselling skills to listen and understand, both the feelings and the relationships; the recipient will feel heard, understood and in a better position to think about the suggestion. But the home care worker will be late for all the other people, some of whom may also have similar needs. On a very practical level it can be difficult to remember what you know from what context and what you are allowed to share. This is one very compelling argument for the provision of supervision for counselling skills users.

Confidentiality

One of the areas of tension in using counselling skills is that of confidentiality. One simple but important way to provide a basic level of confidentiality is to make sure the conversation cannot be overheard. People who use counselling skills in befriending and support agencies will be bound by the codes and policies of the organisation. People who use counselling skills within another primary role are bound by the codes and legal responsibilities of that role with regard to confidentiality. Thus a teacher has limits to the confidentiality that can be offered to pupils. It is important that these limits are made clear before someone starts to confide.

There are other professional boundaries that must be observed and which can be challenging, especially when working in an organisation with colleagues. The counselling skills user may find him/herself taking sides because of what they know, defending someone in ways they would not have done previously and in this way potentially breaching confidentiality.

Referrals

It is important to recognise and accept that when using counselling skills someone may reveal a level of distress that needs more help than counselling skills can provide. In these circumstances, the counselling skills user has a moral responsibility to refer the person to the most suitable help. This requires knowledge of what forms of help are available and how they can be accessed. It is easier to do this, if at the start of the interaction or relationship it has been made clear to the recipient, that if things are beyond your competence, you will suggest a referral.

A pastoral care worker is very clear: 'I know what I can help with and what support I can give, but I've also learnt to recognise when I'm out of my depth. I can listen and support. Sometimes I find out that someone needs more professional help than I can give.'

Over-involvement and boundary setting

In some roles, for example befriending, voluntary work with young people and vulnerable groups and pastoral care, counselling skills users can find it difficult to set boundaries to the support they are willing and able to offer. This can sometimes lead to a feeling of resentment at being 'sucked dry' and expected to be willing and able to listen at any time.

One reason why counselling skills courses devote time to personal development is because seeing the impact of the use of counselling skills can be overwhelming for students. 'It's as if I'd been in another world.' Often students on counselling skills courses want to help others so much, they struggle to accept what they see as 'just listening' and want to offer solutions, make things right. At this stage it is easy to become over involved when trying out the skills: 'If you have no life of your own, then a worry over someone you've seen can worm its way into the centre of your life. It can become difficult to turn off and let go.'

A Trade Union representative became over-involved in a case of bullying at work. He couldn't sleep and found the case taking over his thoughts at work as well. He was able to recognise what was happening and resigned as a union representative.

THE GOOD BITS ABOUT LEARNING AND USING COUNSELLING SKILLS

The previous section is intended to trigger awareness and reflection in anyone training or using counselling skills. But it may have come across as a list of bear traps and pitfalls. This section presents the other side. Counselling skills benefit the user as much as the recipient. For example:

> 'It enabled me to be more assertive.'

> 'I understood my family in a different way.'

> 'I didn't take things so personally after I learnt to listen and try to understand where they were coming from.'

The examples given have already identified some of the roles which can be enhanced by the use of counselling skills. In the extracts below, three people describe how each of them uses counselling skills in very different roles: pastoral worker, customer services officer and university lecturer. These are three of many occupations, in which people regularly choose to use counselling skills.

The pastoral worker blends counselling skills with the faith elements of the job: 'My role is to support people in a spiritual and general wellbeing way, assessing needs, listening and asking questions.' Working with elderly people, often facing the loss of a partner, she finds that using counselling skills enables her to give support in an unobtrusive way. 'I don't feel the need to do anything or sort anything out for them; it is enough that I am there and listening ... I don't get impatient when someone tells me for the sixth or seventh time about the death of their partner. I recognise and understand that they need to do it.' 'Some people just need to be miserable. Me listening to her misery makes her happy in it. There is no wish to change it ... I find that body language and eye contact tell me as much as what is said. Also when I'm leaving I can see that I've been of help, their eyes are brighter.'

The services manager in a charity finds that 'It has made me a better manager. I've learnt to listen to what someone says and let the other person find their own answer, rather than leaping in with suggestions.' In dealing with external people he says 'I have the skills now to be honest and assertive. Before, I would back off if someone was aggressive on the phone, now I know how to respond and I can understand the other person's position better.'

The university tutor finds counselling skills useful in dealing with emotional students: 'I can have an understanding of the emotion but not get drawn into an emotional response, and so I'm able to help the student with the academic consequences of their emotions. For example a student who hasn't handed a piece of work in on time because of family problems, and as result will fail a module. Before, I would have felt under emotional pressure from the student, now I can handle it better.'

A further context in which counselling skills are used is in befriending services such as the Samaritans, Age UK and many others. 'We can help you explore your options and come to your own decisions about what's best for you. Our support may help you find your own way forward.' These words from the Samaritans website, capture the nature and purpose of counselling skills. Services like the Samaritans are staffed by volunteers who undertake in-house training and offer support in a wide range of media, from email to face-to-face meetings. The fact that this is a voluntary activity emphasises the equality between the two parties that is not the case in many of the other examples considered in this chapter. The nurse, teacher, customer services officer, manager all hold some expertise and perhaps authority in their primary role.

COUNSELLING SKILLS TRAINING

The development of counselling skills training courses

As mentioned in Chapter 1, in the 1990s the government of the day introduced National Vocational Qualifications for a wide range of occupations including advice, guidance, mediation, advocacy and counselling. One of the outcomes of this project was the separation and definition of these activities, which included counselling skills. Thus counselling skills were separated from other activities and specific competences were defined and developed into qualifications. The successful completion of a counselling skills course became a route into counselling training.

For many counsellors the first taste of counselling came through attending a course in counselling skills. Counselling skills and introduction to counselling courses are run throughout the United Kingdom. Like counselling courses, counselling skills courses are offered by three kinds of training providers, Registered Awarding Organisations (Credit Rating Bodies in Scotland)[1], Universities and private organisations. The largest numbers of courses are those offered by Registered Awarding Organisations, usually at local colleges of Further Education. The majority of these are courses that offer formal qualifications on the Qualification

---

[1]In Scotland there is the Scottish Credit and Qualifications Framework (SCQF), which is similar to the QCF. This organisation approves organisations which offer qualifications as Credit Rating Bodies. There are currently two CRBs that deliver face-to-face counselling skills and counselling training. These offer formal qualifications on the SCQF.

and Credit Framework (QCF) (Ofqual 2013) (see Table 3.1 on page 45). These QCF registered courses have been reviewed and standardised to a certain extent and are offered by seven Registered Awarding Organisations in accredited centres throughout the country. Tables 2.2 and 2.3 give the outline of the qualifications at Levels 2 and 3. There is usually a progression route to higher level qualifications, often at the same college. The QCF courses have expanded to offer courses at both Levels 2 and 3, often with an expectation that both are needed for progression to counsellor training (Ofqual 2013). This means that following this route to becoming a counsellor will take four to five years.

Courses on the QCF at Levels 2 and 3 will follow the same unit structure and title, but there can be differences in what is taught within the units, as shown in Tables 2.2 and 2.3.

The counselling skills courses offered in Universities may be introductory courses, or may form the first year of a full professional training, with the option to leave at the end of the certificate year. Such a course will include core units such as counselling skills, an overview of the main theoretical approaches, personal development and professional issues. The courses offered by private training organisations tend to be an introduction not just to skills and personal development but also to the particular theoretical approach of the organisation. Such courses may be advertised as, for example, an introduction to humanistic counselling

Table 2.2 *Examples of Level 2 QCF Counselling Skills courses*

Units	Examples of content		
Using Counselling Skills	Identify and practise a range of skills in a counselling skills interaction	Know what counselling skills are	
Counselling skills and personal development	Identify potential source of support	Know how to develop self understanding	
Introduction to counselling skills theory	Key elements of the main theoretical approaches to counselling	Know the three main approaches and how they underpin the use of counselling skills	
Diversity and ethics in the use of counselling skills	Understanding the context in which counselling skills are used. The skills of referral	Concepts of diversity and ethics as applied to the use of counselling skills	Knowledge of discrimination and anti-discriminatory practice

Table 2.3   *Examples of Level 3 QCF Counselling Skills courses*

Unit	Examples of content	Unit	Example of content
Developing counselling skills	How to establish, maintain and end a helping relationship	Developing and practising counselling skills	Set up an effective environment in which to use counselling skills
Theoretical approaches to the use of counselling skills	Know and use key concepts appropriately	Understanding the different approaches to the use of counselling skills	Know the three main theoretical approaches to counselling and what is meant by the integrative model
Working ethically with counselling skills	How to make referrals ethically	Working ethically in a helping relationship	How to relate an ethical framework to the use of counselling skills
Counselling skills and personal development	Explore models of the self and understanding	Understanding the importance of self-development in relation to helping others	Know own development needs
Counselling skills and diversity	How to make referrals		Understand power issues within the counselling process

skills. These courses probably do not give any formal qualification or academic credits. The duration of these courses can be from a weekend to an academic year.

People working in helping professions may find that there are in-house courses or courses approved for career development. If someone is looking for an initial course and may be considering going on to train as a counsellor, it is sensible to take a course that has a clear progression path, either in the same institution or that feeds into a further course at another institution. Voluntary agencies also run their own in-house training which is often about the focus of the agency's work, for example bereavement, domestic violence and available only to staff and volunteers working in the agency.

Counselling skills courses are also offered by distance learning. Counselling skills are learnt and absorbed through practice, experience and feedback. One of the most powerful and effective ways to learn is through group work and practise with other students: distance learning does not give this opportunity.

There is some duplication between counselling skills training courses which overlap with the early parts of counselling training courses. Most counselling skills courses will include the basic listening and responding skills, the values, ethics and attitudes of counselling and an overview of the main theoretical approaches. It is for this reason that most counselling training courses require students to have successfully completed a counselling skills course before starting professional training.

CONCLUSION

Counselling skills can be learnt to be used in their own right and also as a foundation course for entry into counsellor training. People who use counselling skills to enhance other roles are not 'amateur counsellors' or 'would-be counsellors who didn't make it'. Counselling skills users are skilled helpers in their own right. They have chosen a complex and difficult path. Counselling skills users must often hold the values and boundaries of two professions, their primary role and those for counselling skills user. They have to work with a high level of ethical awareness and manage conflicts of interest. The emotional costs can be as great as those experienced by a counsellor, but counselling skills users do not have regular supervision or similar support for this aspect of their work, unless they work as befrienders.

Activities

1 Look at Table 2.1 on page 24. List some of your relationships and see what the balance is. Do any of them look similar to the counselling skills one?

2 List all the reasons why you want to help other people in this way? Do any of them have to do with experiences you have had? Do any of them have to do with what makes you feel good about yourself?

3 Listening and attending. At home, ask someone to help you with this. It takes about 10 minutes. Ask them to talk to you about something ordinary such as holiday plans, or their last holiday. For two minutes give the person your whole attention. For the next two minutes give them an everyday level of attention, the level you may give a partner or child when you are both doing something else at the same time as talking. For the final two minutes give the speaker no attention at all. How did each section feel? What did you notice? You may want to ask the same questions of the speaker.

4 Listening. Make a list of all the things you can think of that can get in the way of you listening to someone. A few have already been mentioned in this chapter.

5 Think about using counselling skills in your current role or with your friends. What concerns do you have? List any possible conflicts of interest. How would you address them?

FURTHER READING

Aldridge, S. and S. Rigby (Eds) (2001). *Counselling Skills in Context*. London, Hodder and Stoughton.

Burnard, P. (2006). *Counselling Skills for Health Professionals*. Cheltenham, Nelson Thornes.

Coles, A. (2003). *Counselling in the Workplace*. Maidenhead, Open University Press/McGraw Hill Education

Culley, S. and T. Bond (2011). *Integrative Counselling Skills in Action* (3rd edition). London, Sage.

Evans, G. (2007). *Counselling Skills for Dummies*. Chichester, John Wiley and Sons.

Geldard, K. and D. Geldard (2003). *Counselling Skills in Everyday Life*. Basingstoke, Macmillan.

Geldard, K. and D. Geldard (2005). *Practical Counselling Skills: An Integrative Approach*. Basingstoke, Palgrave Macmillan.

Hough, M. (2010). *Counselling Skills and Theory*. London, Hodder and Stoughton.

Hutchinson, D. (2102). *The Counselling Skills Practice Manual*. London, Sage.

King, G. (1999). *Counselling Skills for Teachers: Talking Matters*. Buckingham, Open University Press

Linden, J. and L. Linden (2007). *Mastering Counselling Skills*. Basingstoke, Palgrave Macmillan.

McLeod, J. and J. McLeod (2011). *Counselling Skills: A Practical Guide for Counsellors and Helping Professionals*. Second Edition. Maidenhead, Open University Press/McGraw Hill Education

Miller, L. (2011). *Counselling Skills for Social Work*. London, Sage.

Nelson-Jones, R. (2008). *Basic Counselling Skills: A Helpers Manual*. London, Sage.

Rath, J. (2008). 'Training to be a volunteer Rape Crisis counsellor: a qualitative study of womens' experience.' *British Journal of Guidance and Counselling* **36**(1): 19–32.

REFERENCES

Bond, T. (2010). *Standards and Ethics for Counselling in Action*. London, Sage.

Gabriel, L. (2005). *Speaking the Unspeakable: The Ethics of Dual Relationships*. Hove East Sussex, Routledge.

Ofqual (2013). 'Accredited qualifications'. Retrieved 8 May 2013 from www.accreditedqualifications.org.uk.

3   TRAINING IN COUNSELLING

INTRODUCTION

There are so many training courses in counselling on offer, that it is difficult for a prospective student to know which to choose and what to expect. This chapter outlines the current provision of training courses and explains the differences and similarities. It describes the nature and content of typical professional counselling training courses. Many of the elements in counsellor training are the subject of separate chapters in this book. Two that are not, clinical placements and supervision, are covered in this chapter. Finally the chapter identifies the areas for consideration when choosing a training course. The author does not present a consumer guide to training with recommendations; the intention is to provide enough information and questions to enable a potential student to make an informed choice. Trying to present this in a simple clear way has been a challenge, because there is an incoherent complexity to the training courses on offer. The chapter tries to provide some simple information and guidance.

QUALIFICATIONS AND TRAINING IN COUNSELLING IN THE UNITED KINGDOM

There are two national frameworks that set out the levels of formal qualifications awarded in the United Kingdom. These are described below.

The Framework for Higher Education Qualifications (FHEQ) includes all Higher Education University qualifications, that is, degrees at both undergraduate and postgraduate levels. FHEQ courses are delivered by individual Universities. In addition a university may validate the delivery of its courses by Higher and Further Education Colleges and private organisations. Since 2001 a new qualification, the Foundation Degree, a vocational qualification at Level 5 (see Table 3.1), has been available in England, Wales and Northern Ireland.

The Quality Assurance Agency for Higher Education (QAA) oversees the standards of university qualifications and the universities themselves. The QAA produces subject standards, called Subject Benchmark Statements that are linked to the academic framework of higher education qualifications, for example there is a subject benchmark statement for counselling and psychotherapy at undergraduate and postgraduate degree levels (QAA 2013). Qualifications based on the counselling and psychotherapy benchmark statements should 'equip students with the knowledge, skills and experience to practise in therapeutic setting' (QAA 2013).

The second national framework is the Qualifications and Credit Framework (QCF) and the Scottish Qualifications and Credit Framework (SQCF); these cover qualifications that are usually below degree level and are usually described as Diplomas or Certificates. These qualifications are developed and owned by Registered Awarding Organisations that oversee the quality of the courses and award the qualifications.

Ofqual (the Office of qualifications and examinations registration) approves and registers both the Registered Awarding Organisations and the qualifications they offer. The qualifications are usually based on the National Occupations Standards (NOS) for the subject, which have no academic level and many of which are vocational rather than academic. That is, they outline the competences that are required in the subject, for example the NOS for psychological therapies (Fonagy 2010). There are differences in emphasis between the two types of standards, subject benchmarks and NOS. These are outlined in Table 3.2.

Training in such subjects as counselling will include both academic and vocational elements, that is, both theory and practice, if the course aims to produce professional counsellors. The situation is complex – the type of qualification a student gains is not necessarily linked to the type of

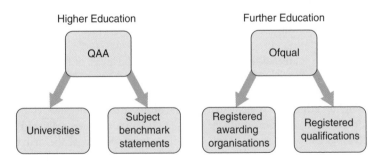

Figure 3.1   *Quality assurance of qualifications*

institution where they studied. For example a private training organisation may deliver a Masters degree from a University; a Further Education College may deliver both a Foundation Degree from a university and a diploma from a Registered Awarding Organisation. In summary, the qualification doesn't necessarily come from the institution where you trained.

Figure 3.1 shows the two main quality assurance systems for educational qualifications in the United Kingdom.

The level of the qualification and what that level means can also be confusing. Table 3.1 provides a read-across table of the qualifications and

Table 3.1   *Qualifications frameworks*

QCF (Qualification and Credit Framework – vocational courses)	FHEQ (Framework for Higher Education Qualifications – courses in universities)	Qualification Level (England, Wales & Northern Ireland)	SCQF Levels (Scottish Qualification and Credit Framework)
Awards and Certificates in counselling skills		2	5
Certificates and Diplomas in counselling skills and counselling studies		3	6
Diplomas in counselling		4	7 Higher National Certificate (HNC)
Diplomas and Higher Level Professional Diploma (HND)	Diploma of Higher Education (Dip HE), Foundation Degree(FD), and Higher National Diploma (HND)	5	8 Higher National Diploma (HND)
	Bachelor Degree (BA, BSc)	6	9/10
	Postgraduate Diploma, Masters Degrees in counselling	7	11
	Doctoral degrees	8	12

levels across the frameworks. There is also a European Qualifications Framework, that I have omitted as this is complicated enough as it is.

The differences in emphasis between the two types of standards, subject benchmarks and National Occupations Standards are indicated in Table 3.2.

Table 3.2   *Comparison between NOS and Subject Benchmark Statement*

Subject	NOS for Psychological Therapies (Roth and Pilling 2011)	Subject Benchmark Statement: Counselling and Psychotherapy (QAA 2013)
Level	None	Undergraduate and postgraduate degree. Levels 6 and 7
Theoretical approach	Cognitive Behavioural, Humanistic, Psychoanalytic/ Psychodynamic and Family and Systemic therapies.	None specified, as applicable to all theoretical approaches.
Emphasis	Emphasis on performance, expressed in the ability to do something. In addition, specific knowledge and understanding that underpins performance.	Emphasis on knowledge and theory and demonstrating conceptual understanding of the theories. Broader abstract concepts.

TRAINING ORGANISATIONS

Traditionally, universities have offered academic courses and Further Education Colleges offer more vocational training. As Table 3.1 shows University courses tend to award higher levels of qualification in counselling than Further Education Colleges. But as already outlined, these boundaries have become blurred especially with the introduction of Foundation Degrees. Private training organisations cannot award any of these nationally recognised qualifications unless the organisation has a formal relationship with a University or a Registered Awarding Organisation which enables them to do this. Such courses will be advertised as validated by a particular university or a Registered Awarding Organisation.

In order to know the type of qualification on offer and its status, prospective students need to read the advertising material very carefully, as Table 3.3 shows.

Table 3.3 *Examples of the advertising information on counsellor training courses – buyer beware!*

Organisation awarding the Qualification	Quality Assurance or Validating organisation	Place training delivered	Title of qualification awarded	Level of qualification awarded	Comment
University of South Riding	QAA	University of South Riding	BA Honours in Counselling	Level 6 on the FHEQ	The qualification is awarded by the University and taught at the University. The level is given as part of the course title. This is a formal nationally recognised qualification.
AQA, a Registered Awarding Organisation	Ofqual	South Riding College	Diploma in Therapeutic Counselling	Level 5 on the QCF	The qualification is one developed by the AQA and validated by Ofqual. It is taught at a college approved by the AQA. This is a formal nationally recognised qualification.
South Riding Consortium	None	At the University of South Riding	Advanced Diploma in Counselling	None. This is a private qualification awarded by the South Riding Consortium	The course has no connection with the University other than the rent it pays to hire rooms. It has no level or formal recognition for its Diploma. The training may be high quality, but it confers no formal nationally recognised qualification.

ROUTES INTO TRAINING

Many people start training by taking an introductory or certificate course in counselling skills. These courses are offered in all the three sectors previously described. Students on these courses will have a range of goals and motivations – to find out more about themselves and how they relate to other people; to enhance interpersonal skills to use in their existing jobs, and as a first step towards a career as a counsellor. Some people will have had experience as a client and wish to 'change sides' as it were. Far more people take counselling skills courses than go on to undertake professional counsellor training.

Counselling skills courses can vary considerably, some are very short, a couple of days or a single term. A more common pattern is a course which runs one evening/afternoon a week over an academic year. Sometimes introductory courses are run at weekends. The courses also vary in content and nature. The introductory counselling skills course is very likely to influence the choices students make about whether or not to continue to professional training and the type of training to move on to.

Introductory courses in the private sector also vary. Many private training organisations offer only one theoretical approach and the introductory course may focus on that approach, rather than give an overview of all the main theoretical approaches. It may be assumed that students who move on to full

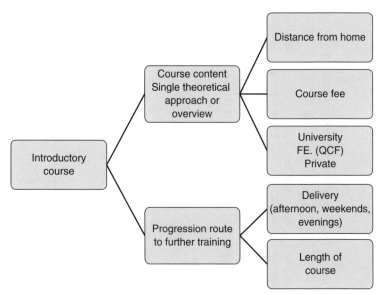

Figure 3.2   *Decision making – introductory course*

training will do so at the same institution. Students choosing such a course need to be sure that this theoretical approach suits them. Some courses will focus on the personal development and self-awareness of the students, rather than give an overview of theoretical approaches on the assumption that the students have already chosen their particular approach. Some private organisations offer short introductory courses as part of the assessment process for entry to full professional training. In others, the introductory course is an essential pre-requisite for full professional training. Others are similar to the QCF and university courses in that they offer a broad introduction to the main theories, counselling skills and personal development.

Figure 3.2 gives some of the elements to think about when choosing an introductory course.

CHOOSING A PROFESSIONAL TRAINING COURSE

What is on offer? There are over 270 counselling courses across the whole of the four home countries. In some areas there will be a great deal of choice in a relatively small geographical area, such as London; in other areas, there will be little choice, for example in the Shetland Islands. Counsellors in Northern Ireland sometimes travel to the Republic, England and Scotland for training. Additional costs in both time and money can restrict choice.

Even if choice is restricted by such factors, it is important to understand what the qualifications on offer mean and what can be expected of a training course. In other words, what might constitute a 'good buy'?

There are several elements a potential student should take into account in choosing a course.

1. The qualification awarded. The most suitable course may not carry the highest academic award.
2. Credibility to employers and the employment outcomes of previous students.
3. Any quality assurance markers, for example recognition by a professional association.
4. Nature of the course – theoretical or practical.
5. Entry requirements.
6. The specific focus in the course, if any – either in terms of theoretical approach or specialist client area.
7. The attendance pattern.
8. Fees and other costs, for example supervision and personal therapy requirements.
9. The arrangements for finding placements.
10. The size of the student intake.
11. The feel of the place.

Table 3.4   *Qualification levels of counselling courses by percentage (BACP 2013a)*

Year	QCF 3	QCF 4	QCF 5	University Dip HE/F. Degree	University BA/BSc	University Postgraduate	None/ Unknown
2013–14	0	25.5	2	17	7	22.4	25
2011–12	0	40	2	23	6	15	13
2010–11	1	36	4	23	7	14	14
2008–09	3	33	3	22	6	12	21

The qualifications awarded

The qualification that is best suited to a student for a range of the reasons given earlier, may not carry the highest academic qualification. In making such a choice potential students need to think carefully about their future career aspirations. If the aim is to work in the public sector, for example, the NHS, it is probably better to choose the highest academic qualification available, as other NHS professions are graduate entry. If a potential student is already a graduate, then it may be sensible to consider

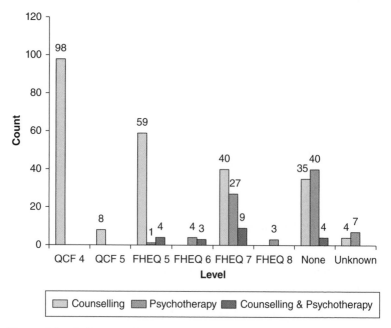

Figure 3.3   *Subject and level of training courses (BACP 2013)*

a postgraduate qualification. A student, who does not plan to become dependent on an income from counselling, has more freedom of choice. However, the most important factor is finding the right course for you. There is a body of research that has tried to identify any correlation between therapists' personality type and theoretical orientation but the outcomes have not been consistent. There has been some correlation between Myers Briggs Type Indicator (MBTI) 'sensing-judgers' and a choice of cognitive behavioural therapy (Topolinski and Hertel 2007; Varlami and Bayne 2007).

Please do not do what I did and stick a pin in a list of courses. My only excuse is that I was living abroad at the time. This was a long time ago and I have been lucky enough to have built a career in counselling.

University training courses   University training courses are offered at both undergraduate and postgraduate level and range from a Foundation Degree or a Diploma in Higher Education, which is normally two years, a full undergraduate degree (a BA or BSc) which is normally three years of full-time study and postgraduate diplomas and Masters degrees which are two to three years part time.

Foundation degrees are awards at Level 5 which are often offered at local Further Education Colleges as well as at Universities. It is a requirement that the University offer a 'top up' year for each of its Foundation Degrees to enable students to gain a full Honours BA or BSc (Level 6). Many counselling training courses in Universities are at Level 5. Every university course will award a formal recognised qualification (see Table 3.1). There is a range of titles used for undergraduate courses in counselling – counselling, counselling studies, counselling and therapeutic studies, therapeutic counselling, theory and practice of counselling, counselling practice. Some courses indicate the theoretical approach taught in the title, for example person-centred counselling. In addition there are joint honours courses which offer counselling with a wide range of other subjects from Media and Communications to IT.

Not all university counselling courses are practitioner training courses; it is difficult to know from the title if the course is a practitioner training course. It is important to make sure that the training course is one which qualifies/equips its graduates to work as counsellors on completion, or it may be necessary to undertake another two–three year training course. It is not always easy to distinguish between these theory-based courses and the practitioner courses, especially not by the course title. Theoretical courses with no practical elements are not practitioner trainings, as they lack the integration of theory with practice through a practicum or clinical placement. Joint honours courses, such as IT with Counselling Studies or Counselling Studies with Law, will not offer a full practitioner training.

Training delivered entirely through distance learning is not accepted as a practitioner training, although it may provide useful professional development for qualified counsellors.

Table 3.5 gives the course outlines of three degree courses in counselling, one of which is not a practitioner training. What is missing is the

Table 3.5 *Comparison of course content*

	Course 1	**Course 2**	**Course 3**
Year 1	Introduction to counselling Counselling skills Psychological and counselling theory Personal development Key issues in counselling	Counselling concepts and skills Concepts in psychology Personal development and interpersonal skills Research methods	Counselling and personal growth The culture of counselling Awareness and communication Coping with change Issues of power and oppression The challenge of individual growth
Year 2	Therapeutic models Counselling skills and theory Preparation for placement Personal development Research methods	Humanistic and Cognitive-behavioural therapy approaches Counselling skills and process Development of the helper Managing diversity in a helping context	Person-centred theory and practice Human development and psychopathology Ethics and professional practice Supervised counselling practice Personal development
Year 3	Placement and supervision groups Professional issues in counselling Counselling settings Mental health and well being	Developing an integrative approach to helping Personal development and career planning Specific issues in helping psychological difficulties	Comparative humanistic counselling approaches Consolidation and integration of professional and personal development
Clinical experience	You will also be supported in arranging relevant work experience to run in parallel with your attendance on the course.	If you choose to undertake some work experience to develop your helping skills in an organisation, the course team will support you to set this up.	Supervised Counselling Practice

integration of theory and practice by means of a mandatory supervised placement. Graduates of Course 2 would need to undertake further two- or three-year training in counselling to become qualified (as the course information states). A student who knows they wish to be qualified to practise would not choose a course of this nature.

QCF qualifications   As shown in Table 3.1 some QCF qualifications in counselling are at a lower level than those offered in universities. This does not necessarily mean that the training is lower quality or less demanding. The fees tend to be lower than university or private training courses. Four Registered Awarding Organisations offer professional counsellor training courses at QCF Levels 4 and 5, with the expectation that where available students will progress from Level 4 to the Level 5 course. One of the advantages of studying for QCF qualifications is that the progression routes are clear and the qualifications are offered throughout Great Britain.

Private training organisations   Private training courses cannot offer a recognised award unless the course has been validated by a university, or the centre and course are accredited by a Registered Awarding Organisation (called a Credit Rating Body (CRB) in Scotland). If the course is university validated this will be indicated in the course brochures and students will be required to pay a registration fee to the university. Private training courses usually advertise the theoretical approaches in the course title, for example psychodynamic training. It may be assumed that the student's choice of the course's particular approach is a deliberate and informed one, when in reality for example, the choice may be more to do with geographical location. Private training providers may not have the range of services and resources available in universities and colleges, for example library, IT facilities, student support services, such as a crèche, learning support, access to loans, and social spaces such as cafes. On the other hand, they may offer a more intimate training space.

Distance learning courses   A search for 'counsellor training courses' on Google will bring up a large number of results, many of which are home study or distance learning courses. These courses are cheap, around £400–£550 and assessed by written assignments. These courses do not meet the training criteria for membership of BACP, which is a one-year full-time or two-year part-time classroom-based counselling or psychotherapy course with a supervised clinical placement of a minimum of 100 hours (BACP 2013b). Some recognised courses deliver what is termed 'blended learning' with certain elements online, but not an entire course.

Credibility of the course

Each year between 3,000 and 4,000 new counsellors qualify from training courses (in addition to psychotherapists and psychologists) and many of them then seek employment and/or set up in private practice. It is therefore a very crowded field. It is useful to find out from the training provider the success of previous students in finding employment. 'Set up in private practice' is not a satisfactory answer, unless this is supported by some evidence that the counsellor actually got clients and did not sit in an empty consulting room until the rent money ran out.

Quality assurance indicators

A training course may hold other indicators of quality assurance, for example it may have been approved or accredited by a professional association. For example, BACP accredits circa 100 training courses (www. bacp.co.uk/accreditation/Accredited%20Course%20Search). Such status indicates that the course has met the standards the professional association considers necessary to produce qualified counsellors (BACP 2012). The professional status of the tutors may also be indicated in course material. Ideally tutors should be qualified and experienced in counselling; this may be indicated by accreditation with BACP or another equivalent professional association.

Entry requirements

Counselling training is very popular and there are often more applicants than places on training courses. The entry requirements are often good indicators when trying to choose a course. There should be a requirement that students have undertaken a substantial introductory course, so that there is some common knowledge within the cohort. Some courses require students to have been in personal therapy before starting the course. Some require students to already have set up a placement for their clinical practice. If faced with either of these last two, the potential student needs to think carefully about whether or not these are reasonable requirements and ask the tutors for the rationale for the requirements before coming to a decision.

Specific focus

Almost all courses will focus on a specific theoretical approach, and students need to be sure that this will suit them. The major theoretical approaches are discussed in Chapter 4. If in doubt, discuss this with the tutor on the introductory course and/or the tutors on the professional training course. Some courses assume that students have previous knowledge and have made an informed choice. For example,

> It is expected that you will have already completed a foundation course that has introduced you to the various orientations, so that the choice of a psychodynamic oriented course is a deliberate and informed one. (www.nescot. ac.uk/higher-education/counselling-/counselling-psychodynamic-diploma-n4610/)

This may present a challenge if you have chosen the course for other reasons, for example it is the nearest or the cheapest.

It may be best to choose an integrative course if uncertain about the theoretical approach (see Chapter 4).

Some courses will train students for work with particular client groups, for example children and young people or people with drug and alcohol issues. Unless a student has experience of such client groups, for example as an Early Years teacher, it is difficult to be certain that such a specialism is the right one, at the start of training. If in doubt students should choose a more general course and specialise later in their career.

Course location and attendance pattern

Such a practical consideration may seem unseemly when debating about one's whole therapeutic future; however, counselling training is often stressful and reducing the sources of stress at the start can only be sensible. Students need to be able to get to and from the course, the placement, supervision and possibly the library. These will all have to be fitted into existing work and family commitments. For many people these practical considerations outweigh all the other factors.

Fees and other costs

Fees vary between courses. Undergraduate university courses are now the most expensive, but some students have access to loans. Postgraduate course fees are very variable and universities charge what they think the market will support. They do not yet appear to have risen in line with undergraduate fees. Private training providers are the next most expensive. If the private provider's course is validated by a University or Awarding Organisation there is an additional fee to that organisation. Qualifications approved by Registered Awarding Organisations have the lowest fees (see Table 3.6).

Table 3.6 *Comparative fees 2012–13*

Training provider	University	University	QCF/Recognised awarding organisation	Private organisation	Private organisation	Private organisation
Course	Undergraduate 3 years full time	Postgraduate 2–3 years part time	Level 4 or Level 5 2–3 years part time	Recognised awarding organisation validated Level 4 or 5 2–3 years part time	University validated Postgraduate 2–3 years part time	No external validation 2–3 years part time
Annual fee	£6,000–£9,000	£2,900–£4,950	£1,500–£1,600	£2,000	£2,500–£3,500	£2,000–£4,500

Other costs   Other costs may include supervision and personal therapy which can add over £4,000 to the cost of training. There will also probably be some residential weekends and some private training organisations require students to pay an annual membership fee of around £50. Many courses require that students join a professional association. The BACP, the foremost association for counselling and psychotherapy in the United Kingdom has a student membership category which costs £70 per annum (£35 reduced) for 2013–14.

Placements/practicum

A practicum or clinical placement is an essential part of counselling training. Students usually begin to work with clients in placements during the second year of training. It can be very difficult to find a placement, especially if there are several counselling training courses in the same town or city. Lack of placement hours is the major cause of delay in completing qualifications. Some courses will arrange placements for students and have a member of staff dedicated to this task. Others run a low-cost service or research clinic in which students can do their placements. Some courses see finding a placement as the responsibility of the student. It is important to discover the attitude and practical help provided by a course before accepting a place. BACP and most training courses do not regard it as safe or ethical for students to do private practice as a training placement. Other aspects of placements are covered later in this chapter.

Size of the training group

This may not be an important factor for some people, but for others it may be important. Very large cohorts can make it difficult to gain enough tutor attention. Very small groups can become difficult if there are relationship tensions within it.

The feel of the place

There is little impartial guidance on this, except to say that, wherever is chosen needs to feel right. A university department and classrooms may feel too cold and academic for the kind of self-exploration undertaken in counselling training. A cosy private course with sofas and cushions and its own cat may hinder the emergence of conflict and challenge for some people. For other people both of these settings may feel safe containing places for such work.

GETTING ONTO A COURSE: WHAT TUTORS LOOK FOR IN STUDENTS

The previous pages have focused on what potential students should look for when choosing a course. This section considers what makes a good student. Given that there are more applicants than places for many courses, it is a good idea to be prepared.

> Training is demanding, intellectually, emotionally and socially. It is not a benign process that can be managed by reading, attending lectures and writing essays, but involves the whole person. (Wheeler, no date)

Counselling training is not an alternative to counselling. The assessment processes used to select entrants for courses are designed to identify anyone looking for therapy rather than for training. The Wolverhampton College prospectus explains this well:

> Counselling practice requires considerable mental stamina and self-awareness and we respectfully remind you that the counselling courses are for training of counsellors and not for personal therapy. We would not recommend anyone to undertake counselling courses within two years of experiencing major personal problems. (www.wolvcoll.ac.uk/course2/tcodp.asp)

Counselling courses are looking for other qualities in potential students and will assess these in the selection processes they hold for potential students. For some private training courses, it appears that a place can be obtained by paying a deposit: 'A deposit of £150 secures a place.'

Selection processes often involve an individual interview and a group experience with other potential students. Tutors are looking for a range of qualities and abilities. Applicants' current level of stability and maturity is a factor; it will be expected that applicants are honest about any previous or current mental health problems. Previous and resolved problems will not be a bar to training, but current problems are likely to raise the issue of a student's resilience to the challenges of training. Life and work experience and the ability to reflect and learn from these is one of the abilities sought, as is the capacity for emotional responsiveness and the ability to relate to others. In addition tutors look for an openness to learning; willingness to take responsibility for that learning and sufficient self-esteem to cope with whatever may emerge.

Some applicants will be rejected; usually this will be because the tutors feel that it is not the right time for the individual to undertake training during which personal vulnerabilities may be exposed, or that the individual would not benefit from the course at that particular time.

THE ELEMENTS IN A TYPICAL COURSE

The curricula of training courses are described in many ways. As already stated there are differences in the way the two national standards describe the subject areas that should be included.

The QAA benchmark statement on counselling and psychotherapy states that 'training is expected to include theory, personal and professional development and competency acquisition' (QAA 2013). In addition the benchmark statement identifies the core components as theoretical input, clinical work, supervision of clinical work, self-awareness and personal development and research skills (QAA 2013: 8). In addition four domains are given:

'A. The professional profile of counselling and psychotherapy:

Professional autonomy and accountability

Professional relationships

B. Maintaining a framework for practice

C. The therapeutic process

D. The social, professional and organisational context for therapy.'

The National Occupational Standards have been developed for four theoretical approaches – cognitive behavioural therapy, psychoanalytic/psychodynamic therapy, family and systemic therapy and humanistic therapy. Within these four approaches are generic competences in addition to theory-specific ones. These are given below:

- Knowledge and understanding of mental health problems.
- Knowledge of an ability to operate within professional and ethical guidelines.
- Knowledge of a model of therapy and ability to understand and employ the model in practice.
- Ability to engage with the client.
- Ability to foster and maintain a good therapeutic alliance and to grasp the client's perspective and 'world view'.
- Ability to deal with the emotional content of the session.
- Ability to manage endings.
- Ability to undertake generic assessment (relevant to history and identify suitability for intervention).
- Ability to make use of supervision.

From these sources it is possible to identify the elements that a course should cover. Most of these have a separate chapter in this book. Placements and supervision are covered in this chapter.

Elements of training courses

1. Theories of counselling, including human development
2. Counselling skills and practice development
3. Personal development
4. Ethical and legal issues
5. Equality and diversity
6. Research and research awareness
7. Placement practice
8. Supervision
9. Personal Therapy

The first five elements are taught within the course, the last three take place outside of the course, although supervision is also a part of practice development and personal therapy contributes to personal development. Personal development, while a separate element, also of course pervades the whole learning process. Although these are presented as separate elements, good training blends them together, which is what a counsellor does in practice. At the beginning of training this can feel like an impossible goal.

When a client makes a statement/says something, the counsellor:

1. Hears what the client is telling them.
2. Attempts to understand what the client is communicating.
3. Attempts to understand what these – the telling, the content and the emotions – mean to the client.
4. Registers the non-verbal communication from the client.
5. Communicates that he/she is fully present with the client.
6. Checks what he/she is selecting to respond to and what is left out; reflects on the reasons for this.
7. Filters what the client is communicating through his/her theoretical approach.
8. Fits the statement within the on-going counselling process with the client and perhaps the client's express goals.
9. Checks own responses and reactions to the client's communication.
10. Frames a response from all of the above.
11. Responds to the client.
12. Is actively aware of how he/she is responding verbally and non-verbally.
13. Is actively aware of how the client responds verbally and non-verbally to the response.

All of this is done in less time than it takes to read the thirteen items. No wonder counsellors respond with quiet fury when counselling is described as 'having a chat' or as something that anyone can do and needs no training.

The skills that are taught are described as counselling or listening skills and many students will have begun such skills training in an introductory course. These skills are extended and used within the theoretical approach of the course. These skills are those needed to create, maintain and end a counselling relationship, to deal with ruptures in relationships. These skills are practised in training on each other so that feedback can be given and acted on without the worry of harming a client. Skills practice provides a safe place to experiment and to begin to integrate theory into practice.

The main difference between a counselling interaction and one with friends is that with friends there is an expectation of a sharing of experiences, feelings etc., but in the counselling relationship the focus is on the client and the counsellor must learn to withhold his/her own views, opinions and desires and try to, as it were, step into the shoes of the client as if they were your own.

As training progresses and students become more confident, students begin to build responses that fit the theoretical approach of the course. Students learn to bring together the skills, knowledge and therapeutic attitudes within a particular theoretical approach and to use this in practice. This may be the focus, the language of responses, and or the way the client communications are understood. It may be the way counselling sessions are structured and the behaviour of the counsellor in the session.

Theory

Chapter 4 outlines the main theoretical approaches and the uses of theory. At the start of practice it is helpful to have a clear theoretical base that provides a solid foundation to refer to, when the new counsellor may feel as lost and confused as the client. Meta analyses of research into the effectiveness of different approaches have shown that no one approach is consistently better than any other. However, research has shown that the counsellor's confidence in the process is a significant variable in positive outcomes (Wampold 2001). In other words, having a theory to use gives confidence. One of the key learning outcomes of training is the ability to link theory to practice. As Kurt Lewin wrote, 'There's nothing so practical as a good theory'(Lewin 1951). Theory helps the counsellor to make sense of a client's concerns and process, as well as their own reactions. During training this ability is developed by retrospective analysis using case discussion groups and case studies of client work.

Ethical and legal issues

This topic is covered in more detail in Chapter 6. All courses will teach ethics; in most counselling courses this will be based on the BACP Ethical Framework for Good Practice in Counselling and Psychotherapy (BACP 2010). It is easy for counsellors to become complacent about these issues, when steeped in the virtues of non-judgemental acceptance and empathy and assume that no further learning is needed.

I fell into this trap when working with a client. One day she turned to me angrily saying, 'How can you ever understand being fat; you're thin!' Indeed I am, and I've been very aware of it and the possible impact of that and all sorts of other aspects of myself ever since. I don't know what it is like to be other than I am.

Research and research awareness

The depth and intensity of training in research and research awareness depends on the qualification. Universities devote more time to this than QCF/SCQF and most private training courses. This topic is covered in more detail in Chapter 7.

Personal development

One of the learning outcomes or goals of counselling training is to develop the ability to be a reflexive/reflective practitioner (Ahern 1999). These two elements combine to help the counsellor develop what is sometimes described as an 'inner supervisor', a rigorous self-questioning/self-searching. This aspect of training and practice is covered in Chapter 5.

CLINICAL PLACEMENTS/PRACTICUM

It may seem to the reader that it is rather odd to have a section on placements, which do not start until at least halfway through training, in a part of the book about choosing a training course. It is here because the placement arrangements need to play a part in choosing a course. Being unsupported by the training organisation in finding a placement can cause immense stress and even withdrawal from the course. For a student the placement is the first real counselling experience and the quality of that placement can make or break a career.

All students on counselling courses are required to have substantial real life experience of counselling clients during training. This is referred to as the 'placement', 'clinical placement' or 'practicum'. The placement usually begins in the second year of professional training, when tutors assess students as ready for practice and continues until the completion of the course or the required number of supervised counselling hours. The required number of hours varies between courses, 100 supervised hours would be the minimum. This can be much harder to achieve than it first appears, as student Chris Molyneux found:

> I entered the placement with a very naïve view that I book 2 clients a week for a year and that's my 100 hours done, no problemo!! I don't think I could have been further from the truth ... (June 2009, www.bacp.co.uk/student/dnas.php)

It cannot be stated often enough, that there are often more counselling students than there are placements, especially in areas with a high density of training courses such as London. Counselling students are also competing for placements with psychotherapy and psychology students. One result of this is that agencies providing placements can be very choosy and make demands on students.

It is not unusual for the placement agency to demand a commitment longer than the duration of the course and to require payment for agency supervision and attendance and payment for in-house training. Some agencies require students to be in therapy for the duration of the placement. Professional indemnity insurance and a Criminal Record Bureau check (£12, 2011) may also be required. Few placements reimburse travelling expenses. Thus students may find that they are paying for the placement.

Finding a placement

Placements, or rather lack of them, are a recurrent theme at meetings of BACP members across the whole of the United Kingdom.

> 'Yes, sorry ... it's a dog eat dog world out there!' she said. I pressed 'end' on my phone and turned to my friend: 'Did you hear that?' It was around the 70th possible placement that we'd contacted. (Perry 2013)

A lucky student will find that their course has a dedicated placement co-ordinator with a good database of agencies and a good track record of successful placements. It is also possible that the training organisation has an in-house service which offers placements. Most students will start with whatever help the training organisation can offer. If a course offers no help or expects students to have placements arranged before the start of training, it may be a good idea to consider alternative courses. A good placement can set the direction of a career.

When applying for a placement it is best to edit the application to reflect the specific focus of the agency, rather than to use one generic application. Agencies may offer set days and hours and students may need to be flexible in what they can offer to gain a placement. Students must abide by the agency's policies and procedures and should ensure that they are made fully aware of these at the start of a placement. This is of great importance for the assessment of client work by the training course.

It may be necessary to have more than one placement to gain the requisite number of client hours. A range of placements can also widen clinical experience and focus career ambitions. It is not unusual for students to carry on in their training placements after completion of the training course to achieve the required number of client hours. If the placement has been half a day a week, with a maximum of three clients, it does not take many DNAs (did not attend) to fall short. Similarly, successful completion of work with a client may leave a gap in the appointment diary. It can be tempting, but unethical, to hang on to clients to get one's hours up!

Features of an ideal placement

Below is a list of the feature that an ideal placement would have:

- The agency has been assessed as suitable by the training organisation.
- There is a formal agreement between the placement agency and the training organisation covering supervision, client hours, the assessment of students and the nature of reports and feedback.
- There is a formal agreement between the student and the placement agency.
- There is a formal agreement over the submission of client work for assessment by the training organisation, covering in particular tape and video recording of client work.
- Agency supervision is provided free of charge. (There is a formal agreement between the supervisor and the placement agency if supervision is external.)
- The placement student has a designated member of staff with whom they meet regularly to discuss caseload and progress and raise concerns if necessary.
- Clients are assessed by an experienced counsellor as suitable for a student's competence and experience and stage of training.
- The agency has a team of experienced counsellors and other students on placement and holds regular meetings for the staff and placement students.
- Placement students have an induction to the agency.
- In-house training and professional development activities are available free to placement students.
- The counselling environment is safe and conducive to the development of therapeutic work. Placement students are never alone in a service.

It should be clear from the above that students should avoid placements in which they are the only counsellor, where they can be at risk of clients beyond their competence with no one to turn to for immediate help. For this reason, among others, private practice is not suitable/acceptable as a placement. Students also need to be aware that some counselling services are in fact networks of independent practitioners who share counselling rooms. These services are not suitable as placements.

SUPERVISION

The training course is the first place that students are likely to have come across supervision. Supervision is a formal relationship between a counsellor and a supervisor within which the counsellor presents his/her client work for discussion. Counsellors in the UK and Europe are required to have supervision throughout their working life. In the USA supervision is seen as necessary only during training and the first years of practice up to licensing. For students in particular supervision provides a way to link theory with practice through the exploration of work with real clients. As Scaife (2009) writes, supervision is a way to get help with the work.

The main purposes of supervision are the welfare of clients and the development of the supervisee's work. This is achieved through the creation of a trusting relationship and safe environment in which learning can take place. In such an environment the supervisee can explore all aspects of client work. There are various forms of supervision (see Table 3.7) and during training students are likely to have some group supervision or case discussion within the course and individual supervision with an external supervisor.

Table 3.7 *Forms of supervision*

Forms of supervision		
1 One supervisor	One-to-one supervision	All clients from all work contexts
2 Several supervisors	One-to-one supervision from each supervisor	Separate supervisor for clients from each context e.g. agency and private practice
3 One supervisor	Group supervision	All clients of all group members. Group may be counsellors from one agency. Number of presentations of client work decided by supervisor and/ or group
4 One supervisor/tutor	Case discussion group	Focus of client presentation. Number and type of presentation decided by supervisor/tutor
5 Shared responsibility	Peer group supervision	Clients of all group members. Number of presentations of client work decided by group

Supervision contracts

Supervision needs to be formally contracted. In the case of students, this will be a three-way contract, with the supervisor having responsibilities to the training course, in addition to the supervisee and his/her clients. Contracts should include practical elements such as location, length and frequency of sessions, fees, emergency contacts and any assessment or reporting on the quality of the supervisee's practice. The methods of presenting client work should be agreed at the start, such as verbal presentation, notes, tape recordings etc. It is also worth discussing the options if things should go wrong, the ethical responsibility of the supervisor to report poor practice and the limits of confidentiality. Both parties will have implicit expectations of the other and it is a good idea to try to make these more explicit. For example, the supervisor may be very well known and respected and the student supervisee may feel terrified at the prospect of revealing his/her work to such an eminent person.

How much is enough? This question has no correct answer in terms of number of hours or frequency. The answer is whatever enables the counsellor to feel professionally and personally supported in all their work. Students benefit from more supervision rather than less, and this is often built into course requirements, with a mixture of external and internal supervision and case discussion. BACP counsellor/psychotherapist accreditation requires 1.5 hours a month and some employers have adopted this.

The supervision of students

Both supervisor and supervisee have responsibilities in the relationship, but it is more difficult for the student at the start of the career to recognise this mutuality, especially if the supervisor has some formal assessment responsibility. There is evidence to suggest a better working alliance if the counsellor has a choice of supervisor, than if one is allocated. Both have a responsibility to work to the contract and to review this regularly.

The supervisor must work in a way that is consistent with the course approach; to do otherwise will confuse and undermine students' confidence. The supervisor needs to be very clear and open with the student about the obligations to the course and any assessment or evaluation involved. Students can fail to present difficult clients and errors if they fear that these will be reported back to the course. The supervisor must try to create a relationship that will mitigate such fears and foster the development of confidence and competence. The supervisee has a responsibility to be honest and open to learning and to take back to practice insights and learning gained in supervision. Support and education are the two most important elements in the supervision of students.

There are many common elements in supervision which are outlined below. Differences arising from the theoretical approaches are covered in Chapter 4. The common elements can be summarised as:

1. What happened in the session(s) and how. That is content and techniques and interventions.
2. The supervisee–client relationship, both in the session and in the supervision. That is the feelings evoked by the client in the session and during supervision.
3. The supervisor–supervisee relationship in the here and now of the supervision session. This may elicit a parallel process where the supervisee enacts the dynamic between him/herself and the client with the supervisor.
4. An increased theoretical understanding as the link between theory and practice becomes clear.

For example, a supervisee may find the supervisor indifferent and even critical when discussing a client who fears rejection in relationships. Exploration of the possibility of a parallel process enables the supervisee to see that he has been caught in replaying the client's pattern of relationships by being distant and cold with the client. This insight will help the supervisee understand better the client's world view and use this positively in the relationship (adapted from Aveline 2007).

Research has identified some aspects of supervision and supervisors that are positive and some that are negative. Poor supervisory practice does not focus on the supervisee's story or concerns, or on the here and now of the session. Poor supervision is not supportive or affirming; it may be hostile and critical. Supervisees in such supervision are unlikely to reveal fears and anxieties about poor practice. Some research suggests that such poor supervision arises from lack of training and experience or a poor fit with the approach of the supervisee.

Good supervision will have a mutually agreed contract that is subject to review and evaluation and a strong therapeutic alliance and secure attachment (Foster et al. 2007). This will enable the supervisee to feel confident to disclose difficult practice and learn how to deal with such things as negative feelings about clients. The supervisor will allow the supervisee to give an account of the work and closely track the concerns and queries. He/she will respond to specifics rather than generalities. Good supervision helps the student to learn and to feel confident in the work.

A poor experience of supervision in training can have a lasting negative impact. It is better to change supervisor than to stay in a relationship where little learning is taking place. Good supervision will support and expand knowledge and competence throughout a counsellor's working life.

CONCLUSION

This chapter has outlined the choice of training courses and the elements that comprise counsellor training. It is hoped that this will increase the chance of readers making a more informed choice and have some idea of what to expect during training.

When choosing a course, even if you have no real choice for reasons of fees and location, potential students need to be aware that starting a counsellor training course is not the same as starting a history or physics degree. The student will be buying into the ideology of the theoretical approach and will be socialised into its philosophy and values. The student will learn a new language, gain a new family and learn that family's table manners and idiosyncrasies. He/she is likely to become an adherent/follower of that approach, at least in the first few years of practice. Someone starting out on the two- to three-year training process will not be the same person at the end.

REFERENCES

Ahern, K. J. (1999). 'Ten tips for reflexive bracketing.' *Qualitative Health Research* **9**: 407–11.

Aveline, M. (2007). 'The training and supervision of individual therapists'. In W. Dryden, *Dryden's Handbook of Individual Therapy*. London, Sage: 515–48.

BACP (2010). *Ethical Framework for Good Practice in Counselling and Psychotherapy*. Lutterworth, BACP.

BACP (2013a). *Training Map 2013–14*. Lutterworth, BACP.

BACP (2013b). 'An invitation to membership.' *Application Pack*. Lutterworth, BACP.

Fonagy, P. (Ed.) (2010). *Digest of NOS for Psychological Therapies*. Bristol, Skills for Health.

Foster, J.T., J.W. Lichtenberg and V. Peyton, V. (2007). 'The supervisory relationship as a predictor of the professional development of the supervisee.' *Psychotherapy Research* **17**(3): 343–50.

Lewin, K. (1951). *Field Theory in Social Science*. New York, Harper.

Perry, M. (2013). 'From out of the frying pan.' *Therapy Today* **24**(3): 8.

QAA (2013). *Subject Benchmark Statement. Counselling and Psychotherapy*. Gloucester, Quality Assurance Agency for Higher Education.

Roth, A. and S. Pilling. (2011). 'Competence Framework for the delivery and supervision of psychological therapies.' Retrieved 26 April 2013, from www.ucl.ac.uk/clinical-psychology/CORE/competence_frameworks.ht.

Scaife, J. (2009). *Supervision in Clinical Practice: A Practitioner's Guide.* Hove East Sussex, Routledege.

Topolinski, S. and G. Hertel (2007). 'The role of personality in psycho-therapists' careers: Relationship between personality traits, therapeutic schools and job satisfaction.' *Psychotherapy Research* **17**(3): 365–75.

Varlami, E. and R. Bayne (2007). 'Psychological types and counselling psychology trainees' choice of counselling orientation.' *Counselling Psychology Quarterly* **20**(4): 361–73.

Wampold, B. E. (2001). *The Great Psychotherapy Debate: Models, Methods and Findings.* Mahwah, NJ, Erlbaum.

Wheeler, S. (no date). Retrieved 26 May 2012 from ww2.le.ac.uk/departments/lifelong-learning/counselling

4 THEORETICAL APPROACHES TO COUNSELLING

INTRODUCTION

Counselling is usually described as 'counselling' without any adjective indicating a particular theoretical approach. In contrast, psychotherapy and psychoanalysis usually indicate the particular theoretical approach – for example 'psychodynamic' psychotherapy or 'cognitive behavioural' psychotherapy. This has led to a mistaken belief that counselling has no underpinning theory and is little more than a set of interpersonal skills; a belief reinforced by the fact that in counselling training, skills are identified and specifically taught whereas in traditional psychotherapy it is assumed these skills will be acquired without training. Another mistaken assumption is that counselling is restricted to the humanistic theories. To set this straight: all counsellors study at least one theoretical approach in depth, across the whole range of theories.

This chapter outlines the uses of theory to the counsellor and gives a brief overview of four theoretical approaches: psychoanalytic/psycho dynamic, cognitive behavioural, humanistic, including person-centred and integrative. All these approaches have been written about in more detail and a selected reading list is provided in the bibliography. The aim is to help prospective students and clients to make informed choices about theoretical approaches.

There are said to be over 400 separate approaches in counselling and psychotherapy. Whether or not this is the case, the four major groups listed above are the best known. They represent the most common counselling approaches taught and practised in the United Kingdom at present. New approaches have and continue to develop, for example Cooper and McLeod's pluralism (2011). Looking at the counselling theory books published in the 1960s and 1970s it is clear that many had a very short life, often coinciding with that of the charismatic founder of the approach.

WHAT IS A 'THEORETICAL APPROACH' OR A 'THEORY' OF COUNSELLING?

This section looks at the uses and usefulness of theory in counselling. There are many debates and arguments over theories of counselling and psychotherapy; adherents claim better outcomes for their particular theory. Some claim that only strict adherence to a manual of treatment for a specific disorder will bring about a positive outcome. Others argue that matching the type of intervention to the client's changing presentation and experience within therapy will bring about a positive outcome. Some theories argue for open-ended long-term work, others use research to show that the main changes occur in the first three sessions.

Given the level of disagreement between the theories on such important issues one might ask if it is necessary to have theories of counselling. Whether, theories of counselling provide anything more than a platform from which to argue with other counsellors?

Each theoretical approach to counselling is based upon a particular set of beliefs about how we become ourselves. In more theoretical language, this would be described as theories on human development and the ways in which psychological, emotional and relational problems develop and are maintained. Thus each approach has an underpinning set of philosophical beliefs about the nature of human beings and the meaning of life. Each approach also promotes the ways in which its interventions and techniques are used to aid clients to address such difficulties. It is believed that when a theoretical approach is used properly it will result in a good client outcome. Not surprisingly, all theoretical approaches believe in their effectiveness with clients. The scientific method of theory development is to develop a hypothesis and test it scientifically to produce a theory to explain cause and effect. Many counselling theories have not been developed in this way, but derive more from a body of ideas arising from observation and explanation of clients' processes. These may then be used as a basis for research to test hypotheses.

THE USES OF A THEORETICAL APPROACH

In simple terms, a theoretical approach provides a map or guidebook, to be used for reference on the journey that is the counselling process. There are many other metaphors for the use and purpose of theory. Theory gives the counsellor the following:

- A way of understanding human development and behaviour.
- A rationale for the development and progress of the problems that bring people into counselling.

- A way of understanding how and why change might occur.
- Ways in which to work with clients to address these problems and issues.
- A map of what might happen in the counselling process.
- Theory offers guidance to the counsellor on how to behave in the counselling process, in terms of building the therapeutic relationship, or delivering a manualised set of interventions.
- It is a language to use to communicate all of the above to oneself, the client and colleagues.

In training, theory provides a structure within which to learn and practise. Research has shown that newly qualified counsellors work closely within the theoretical approach of their training; more experienced therapists tend to develop a unique blend of theoretical approaches (Skovholt and Ronnestad 1992). At the start of practice it is helpful to have a clear theoretical base which provides a solid foundation to refer to, when the new counsellor may feel as lost and confused as the client.

Figure 4.1 shows three separate but overlapping elements – content, context and process – which are essential to professional practice and the transferability of learning between these elements. These elements are in constant interplay from the start of training and throughout professional practice (Rosen 2012: 14).

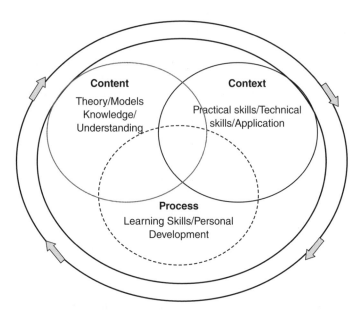

Figure 4.1   *The elements of professional practice*

All counselling courses contain theory and all counsellors use at least one theoretical approach in their work. The tendency to focus on a single theoretical approach in training is a somewhat unusual way to deliver education. In many disciplines, students are encouraged to explore and critically analyse alternative models or hypotheses. The narrow focus arises from the history of the talking therapies. More recently the evidence prioritised in the development of National Institute for Health and Care Excellence (NICE) guidelines, has also favoured the adoption of a single theoretical approach (see Chapter 7 on Research).

Students are socialised to be loyal to the theoretical approach and its superiority over other approaches. This process is somewhat similar to conversion and adherence to a particular belief system.

Sometimes this is overtly communicated, for example until quite recently graduates of British Psychoanalytic Council courses were forbidden to belong to any other professional association. Sometimes it is more implicit. Some counsellors stay with the theoretical approach of their original training throughout their working lives, while others widen the theoretical base through further training. Whichever path is taken, the blend of training and experience and professional development results in each counsellor creating his/her unique integration of personality, theory and practice.

McLeod (2009) suggests that the different theoretical approaches may be understood as different languages all talking about the same thing. But just as the English language for example has several sorts of 'pink', other languages may have only one word such as the Danish 'light red'. Translation is not always easy. A story with a beginning, middle and end is very reassuring to a student and novice counsellor.

Let us use the metaphor of counselling approaches as a set of maps; maps come in a variety of formats and use a range of symbols. Some symbols may be common to several maps. The student user must select the map they find easiest to read and understand; the one that will help them most on the journey. They must then learn to read it and transfer the knowledge and understanding into the landscape of the counselling session.

HOW TO CHOOSE A THEORETICAL APPROACH

As already mentioned in Chapter 3 on training, in reality choice may be restricted to what is available locally and what is affordable. However, if choice is an option, how is the choice made? It is possible that a theoretical approach will be in conflict with a student's own beliefs and value systems, for example, someone who believes in the doctrine of original sin may struggle with the person-centred belief in human potential and self-actualisation, with its underpinning belief in free will. Whilst challenging assumptions is an essential part of training, challenging a student's core beliefs and value systems must be done sensitively. Too great a challenge during training can be harmful. Dogmatic or over-assertive challenges present a poor model of practice. Some research suggests that certain personality types fit better with certain theoretical approaches and that a 'bad fit' can have a negative effect on the counsellor and client outcomes (Topolinski and Hertel 2007; Varlami and Bayne 2007).

Each theoretical approach has a clear concept of what constitutes a good therapeutic outcome. Underneath these are powerful value systems and belief structures that are culturally derived. One criticism made of many counselling theories is that they come from the American and European individualistic cultures, with Western models of relationships. It is worth noting that most of the founders of theoretical approaches were men living in Western society and culture and the theories and treatments must be seen and understood in that social and economic context. Feminist therapy developed as a response to this as part of the women's movement from the late 1960s (Brown 2010). It is enlightening to look at each counselling approach in the context of the social and economic conditions prevalent when it was developed and the personal circumstances of the founder. For example, there is a body of critique of psychoanalytic therapy that sees it as bound by the patriarchal attitudes and values of nineteenth-century middle European culture and the subordinate position of women in that culture (Masson 1990). Other cultures have their own ways of understanding and addressing psychological distress.

THE MAJOR THEORETICAL APPROACHES

The origins of theoretical approaches

This section presents a very brief overview of the origins and features of four major theoretical approaches. A more detailed overview of a greater range of approaches can be found in Dryden and Reeves' *Handbook of Individual Therapy* (2014).

The ideas from which the talking therapies emerged began with the creation of psychoanalysis by Freud and Breuer in nineteenth-century Vienna. Psychoanalysis marked a new way to understand and treat mental illness and distress, by locating the origins within the individual and explaining mental illnesses and distress as the outward signs of unconscious internal intra-psychic conflicts. While this is a massive over-simplification, the important principle that was carried into other approaches is that human distress and psychological problems can be expressed through physical symptoms and that talking in a formal setting to an interested third party (therapist) can help.

Behaviour therapy emerged from a very different home, based in observation and experimental testing of theories of behaviour change, originally with animals. Cognitive Behavioural Therapy (CBT) arose from the combination of elements of Behaviour theory with Beck's theories of cognition and Ellis's theory of underlying belief systems. Psychoanalysis and Cognitive Behavioural Therapy were the two recognised theoretical approaches found in the United Kingdom until the second half of the twentieth century.

The range of theoretical approaches that are bracketed together as Humanistic came to prominence in the USA and UK in the 1960s and 1970s. Perhaps the best known of these is Person-Centred counselling, developed by Carl Rogers in the USA in the 1940s and 1950s. The Humanistic theoretical approaches can be understood as reaction and opposition to the two established models. Certainly the humanistic values were more in keeping with the culture of the period.

A fourth group fall under the title of 'integrative' (Holmes and Bateman 2002). Reference to an integrative theoretical model can be misleading, as there are several models of integration. Some seek to integrate two or more theoretical approaches and as such do not create a new theoretical approach. Others have developed a process model and fit interventions from various theories into the process. Others use research into the variables which make counselling effective to identify the common factors found in all theoretical approaches. This range of integrative approaches is discussed in more detail later in this chapter. Eclecticism was an approach used before integrative: this involved the selection of an intervention from a range of theories, which seemed to best fit the client at that particular moment for the particular issue, for example Egan's Skilled Helper (1975).

The diversity of theoretical approaches has led to dispute and disagreement over which, if any, is right or produce better outcomes for clients. Proponents of Psychoanalysis and Behavioural Therapy fought a very public battle in the 1950s and 1960s over claims to be scientific (Eysenck 1952). Currently CBT has been fighting a similar battle with all other theoretical approaches using its scientific background and Randomised Controlled Trials as evidence of greater effectiveness (see Chapter 7 on Research).

SUMMARY OF THE MAJOR APPROACHES

Most theoretical approaches have a view of the nature of human beings, the reasons why people develop psychological difficulties and ideas about what might help bring about change, reduce or remove the difficulties. All approaches explain the processes of change, and the role of the counsellor in this process.

Some approaches focus on specific problems or conditions, such as anxiety or post-traumatic stress. In these approaches the focus is on interventions which are used systematically with clients to remove the symptoms. Success is measured by a reduction in symptoms and the development of strategies to prevent or deal with recurrence. Other approaches work with the whole person of the client and take into account the context such as family, cultural, social and economic factors. While these approaches have some specific interventions, there is an emphasis on the relationship between the client and counsellor – the therapeutic alliance, which is seen as a significant factor in good client outcomes. More recently, research has identified 'common factors' which are found in all approaches and this is one of the reasons for the rise of 'integrative theories' (Wampold 2001; Drisko 2004; Roth and Fonagy 2006).

It is possible to see a division in the theories between positivist approaches, those which believe that they are the 'truth', and the postmodern approaches that use theories as a way of subjectively understanding people and problems. Psychoanalytic/psychodynamic theories have been described as pessimistic in their view of human beings as constantly fighting internal conflicts; whilst humanistic theories are seen as more optimistic with the belief in human potential, given the right conditions. Whichever theoretical approach is taken, 'there is unequivocal evidence that, on average, psychological therapies have a positive effect on people's mental health and wellbeing' (Cooper 2008: 34). This contrasts with Smail's argument that therapy cannot cure the social and environmental conditions that are the causes of distress; at best all any approach can do is offer comfort (2001).

PSYCHOANALYTIC/PSYCHODYNAMIC APPROACHES

Psychoanalysis is the name given to the 'talking therapy' developed by Freud in nineteenth-century Vienna. There were early divisions within the group around which led to the founding of other theoretical approaches such as those of Jung, Ferenczi, Reich and Adler, and later Klein and Anna Freud. Today there is considerable theoretical diversity and theories are more likely to be described as psychodynamic and be identified by the name of the founding figure, e.g. Jungian psychodynamic psychotherapy. Some of the practices of these early analysts would be greeted today with horror. It was not unusual for a psychoanalyst to send his wife to a colleague for analysis and discuss her progress with him (Maddox 2006).

Psychodynamic counselling in the United Kingdom uses the psycho-analytic theories of Freud, Jung, Klein and Anna Freud, and the later theoretical developments of, for example, Bowlby and Winnecott. Freud and his colleagues, in particular Breuer, developed the theory that the symptoms shown by patients were the expression of internal conflicts of which the patients were unaware. These unconscious conflicts were brought into conscious awareness through analysis, by means of free asso-ciation and recall of dreams.

Freud believed that sexuality was one of the major areas of internal conflict which was put out of conscious awareness to protect the child from unbearable anxiety in the face of the conflicting desires. Some later theorists have moved away from such focus on infant sexuality. These intra-psychic conflicts appear later in life through physical symptoms, such as hysteria, anxiety and psychosomatic illness – that is psychologi-cal illness which has physical symptoms, without any organic/physical cause. This may include self-harming and other self-destructive self-limiting behaviour. These inner conflicts are kept unconscious by 'defence mechanisms' such as repression and resistance. Defence mecha-nisms are the ways in which we protect ourselves from the full force of the internal conflicts and unacceptable desires, which would otherwise be unbearable. In the United Kingdom in some theoretical schools there has been more focus on the transference relationships between counsel-lor and client.

Psychodynamic /psychoanalytic theories share some common assump-tions. These are that individuals are conditioned by experiences with early care givers and that these relationships tend to influence behaviour in relationships in adult life. More recent theoretical developments believe that later attachments (relationships) can lead to change in the pattern of relationships set in childhood.

These approaches saw the relationship with the therapist as the space in which the unconscious becomes conscious. Clients reveal these dysfunc-tional relationship patterns by re-enacting these in the relationship with the psychoanalyst (transference). Transference means that the client reacts/responds to aspects of the counsellor, as if he/she was a significant person from their past. The counsellor is able to use the transference relationship to gain understanding of the client's problems. Later theoretical develop-ments gave attention to the counsellor's transference towards the client (counter-transference). That is, that the counsellor might react to the cli-ents as if he/she was a significant person from the counsellor's past. This is one of the reasons for the requirement for personal therapy or analysis for students, to enable them to bring their transference reactions and intra-psychic conflicts into conscious awareness and address them if necessary rather than responding to these unconscious urges when working with clients.

Psychoanalytic theory presupposes that we do not have random thoughts or reactions; our reactions have been conditioned by earlier events and experiences. It follows therefore that all our thoughts and behaviours have a purpose, even if we are not consciously aware of that purpose. Some early experiences are so distressing that they are kept out of conscious awareness. This does not necessarily mean that the experiences were traumatic in a tabloid newspaper way, but that they were traumatic and distressing to the baby or small child.

For example: for years, I could not sleep with a picture on the wall above the bed. I had nightmares. In hotel rooms I would pull pictures down in my sleep and find them on the floor in the morning. One day, my mother recalled how I had embarrassed her when I was a baby. A nun had bent over the pram to look at me and I had screamed and howled until the poor woman moved away. My nightmares stopped immediately, as what had been repressed and unconscious was made conscious and I didn't need to be afraid anymore.

Developments in psychodynamic theory led to a change in perception from Freud's view of human beings as biologically driven to human beings as social beings, who needed secure attachments to other people. Bowlby's (1979) attachment theory argues that human beings need the experience of early secure attachments in order to function well in later life.

Freud's ideas have been subject to scrutiny and critique; however, many of his ideas form the basis of modern psychodynamic theory. Three theoretical concepts remain at the core: that an individual's problems originate in formative experiences, however unclear the connection; the individual is not aware of the motives for his/her behaviour; the importance of the use of transference in the therapeutic relationship. The goal of the analysis is greater insight, which may not necessarily lead to change.

Jung did not share Freud's view that an individual's personality is fixed in early childhood; he believed people continued to develop throughout life. Central to Jung's approach is the concept of opposites, both in individuals and cultures. In the individual, psychological distress or neurosis results from taking a position at one of the extremes. The aim of therapy is to find a way to hold the balance between the opposites. Jungian theory has widened this idea to conceptualise 'opposites' more as a range of possibilities. Jung's view of the unconscious differed from that of Freud; he theorised the psyche as both the personal and also the collective unconscious of archetypes, which represent universal aspects of human experience both positive and negative. The aim of therapy is to enable the client to attain a state of wholeness by synthesising opposite forces. Jung saw the search for self-knowledge as spiritual and this and the mystical elements of his theories have not fitted well into the current demand for evidence-based therapies (Casement 2007). From Jung's theory of innate personality types we have taken into everyday life the concept of introvert and extrovert and the Myers-Briggs personality typing instrument. Jung also contributed to the idea of the therapist as a 'wounded healer'; the idea that we may be attracted to a helping profession to primarily meet our own needs (see Chapter 5). Jung and others have suggested that the therapist can use their vulnerabilities to positive effect (Sedgwick 1994).

Originally the analyst/therapist was inactive in the relationship to allow the client's transference to emerge. Classic psychoanalysis puts the client on the couch and the analyst sits behind the client out of sight to enable the client to free associate. The analyst makes interpretations from time to time. Some approaches now give the therapist a more active role in the relationship and the couch has sometimes been replaced by a chair.

Criticisms of psychoanalytic/psychodynamic theory

Perhaps one of the best known criticisms would be better described as an outright attack: Hans Eysenck (1952) published a paper that showed that psychoanalytic psychotherapy did not lead to recovery from neurotic disorders. Within this was the criticism that psychotherapists based outcome evaluation on 'subjective certainty' rather than 'objective facts' (Eysenck 1952). That is, psychoanalysis is unscientific and opposed to research. The psychoanalysts' response is that each patient constitutes research. One issue is the power of the therapist which is enhanced by the pre-eminence given to the transference interpretations. It is argued that this emphasis on the development of the transference encourages the dependence and vulnerability in the client. This gives the therapist immense power over the client. Masson argues that psychotherapy is an abuse of power, in which the therapist forces interpretations on the client. A lack of acceptance of an interpretation is evidence of resistance or repression, not of an inaccurate or insensitive interpretation by the therapist (1990). A more down-to-earth observation is that the whole process takes too long and produces 'converts not cures'. Psychoanalysis, several times a week, is expensive and as a result inaccessible to many people. Clients can experience the relationship as cold: one client was left feeling insignificant, 'less than nothing' when at the end of six years of therapy his analyst did not acknowledge that the relationship was ending.

Psychodynamic/psychoanalytic theories are viewed as pessimistic: human beings are seen as capable of self-deception, driven by internal conflict over unacceptable desires and strong emotions, with little conscious control over their expression in everyday life and relationships. It is also argued that because the goal of therapy is insight not behaviour change, it might reinforce destructive relationship patterns and behaviour.

COGNITIVE BEHAVIOURAL THERAPY

Cognitive Behavioural Therapy (CBT), as its name suggests, is more than one approach. It is a pragmatic theoretical approach and has consistently added and developed other approaches if they can be proved to be effective, and continues to do so. CBT began to be developed in Britain in the 1960s and 1970s at the Maudsley Hospital in London. Behaviour therapy originated in theories of behaviour modification, mainstream experimental psychology and learning theory. As a result the theoretical approach incorporates the scientific methods of experimentation and seeks reliable and observable, that is, evidence-based, outcomes. Theories on cognitions or thinking/thoughts were added to behaviour modification theories in an attempt to get a better understanding of psychological problems. This combination is used as a base for a theory of the origins and treatments of psychological problems. A central belief is the need to identify and change unhelpful thoughts and behaviours.

CBT therefore, began with a scientific rationale, firmly based in experimentation, observation and evidence-based techniques. CBT is based on what can be observed, studied and reliably measured, and this has led CBT to focus on specific conditions or illnesses, conditions evidenced by the beliefs an individual holds which affect both their behaviour and emotions, rather than the whole person. Thoughts and meaning can be identified and changed and this will result in changes in behaviour and feelings. In CBT the client can experiment with changing thoughts and observe his/her behaviour for changes at the same time.

One of the main ideas taken from behaviour modification is that of the cycle of stimulus and response, and how response experienced as a reward will reinforce the behaviour thus rewarded. This can result in self-defeating and self-limiting patterns being rewarded and thus reinforced in clients. This means that we will continue to do something if it is rewarded, even if the reward may not appear to be such to an outside observer.

Cognitive theory (Ellis 1994) suggests that people need to construct meaning and use such meaning to manage their life. For example, someone may believe that worrying stops bad things happening, so it becomes necessary to worry if a partner is late home. When the partner arrives home safely, this proves that the worrying worked! In order to change this, the individual will need to change the meaning they give to worrying. In summary, if the meaning can be changed then the behaviour and feelings will also change as a consequence. A further contribution which has influenced CBT in this country is Beck's (1976) proposition that individuals have beliefs which are expressed as automatic thought processes. In order to address these, the theory requires attention to specific details and symptoms in order to develop a detailed treatment plan. In CBT these patterns of thinking and feeling are called 'schema' and 'formulations'.

The key principles in CBT are the need for the active engagement of the client, and the focus on symptom removal and strategies to deal with recurrences. A client entering CBT must actively engage and be motivated to work on the problems and possible solutions both in and between sessions. This focus on the specific and detailed aspects of the problem with the active engagement of the client can instil hope and a sense of achievement. The active collaboration appears to deal with the issues of resistance and defence mechanisms. The client must focus on the removal of his/her symptoms and the development and testing of strategies to do this and prevent recurrence. The relationship between counsellor and client is recognised as important: it is a task-focused relationship in which both parties focus on the client's goals and how to achieve these.

Criticisms of CBT

CBT is criticised as paying little or no attention to the therapeutic relationship, and as being too task-focused. While it is recognised that a good working relationship contributes to the achievement of good client outcomes, there is little attention to the therapeutic relationship itself as a vehicle for client change. It is argued by critics that the focus on symptom removal and on specific conditions ignores the person and treats the client as an object. One person had had CBT for an irrational fear that was controlling her life. She was relieved that she had been helped to overcome the fear, but wanted to understand the origins of that reaction and whether this was related to her past or her family. It is also argued that the removal of symptoms and the creation of strategies to deal with the recurrence of symptoms do not address the underlying causes of the distress. This focus on specific disorders can lead to the labelling of ordinary misery and unhappiness as mental illness rather than it being seen as part of ordinary life. One counsellor colleague was shocked to see a leaflet in her General Practice suggesting that someone who was still feeling grief six weeks after losing a life partner should see the doctor about CBT treatment for depression.

HUMANISTIC APPROACHES

This group of theoretical approaches developed in the second half of the twentieth century as a reaction to both Cognitive Behavioural Therapy and Psychoanalysis. The many different theories have in common an acceptance of ordinary life and the common human issues of life, death, relationships, hope and how we make sense of these. This means that subjectivity is respected in the Humanistic approaches, the way in which each of us makes sense of the world in our own way. The human being is seen as a whole, within a current social, economic and cultural context, rather than as a set of symptoms. The philosophical beliefs take a positive view of human beings, given the right conditions; thus people can grow and achieve their potential. People are seen as strong, capable of self-determination, held back from achieving potential by negative experiences in the family or dominant culture.

There is a wide range of approaches; some are taught and practised under a discrete theoretical name, such as Person-Centred Counselling, Gestalt Therapy, Transactional Analysis, Transpersonal Therapy. The goal of counselling is for the client to be able to recognise their potential; in order to do this the client must accept him/herself. The counsellor's acceptance of the client is a key therapeutic element in this process. The aim is for the client to learn that he/she has the capacity to change and improve their quality of life. Change is not necessarily the goal of humanistic counselling in the way that it is in CBT.

Humanistic theories have a positive view of people and make no division between person and problem. The view of humans as social beings supports the belief in the healing power of the therapeutic relationship between counsellor and client. Humanistic theories recognise that each of us constructs meaning in our lives in the best way possible. Humanistic counsellors use these meanings to help the client realise their potential. The relationship with the counsellor, is the space in which the client experiences acceptance and is supported to explore the meanings and potential of their life.

Humanistic approaches identify the importance of 'real' experience in the development and treatment of psychological problems and the reparative power of the 'here and now' real contact between the counsellor and client. This relationship is the heart of therapy. Therefore the goal of humanistic therapy is to create in the relationship a form of therapy which will work for both parties – counsellor and client. The emphasis is on the relationship between client and counsellor in the present, the here and now. This is contrasted with the transference/counter-transference relationship of the psychoanalytic/psychodynamic approaches, which represent a replaying of old relationship patterns. However, the behaviours of counsellor and client are probably the same, but understood differently.

Existential counselling, while sitting within the Humanistic school, has different roots to the other counselling theories. It developed from European philosophy and aims to help the client to find meaning in life and to take responsibility for choices made. Existential therapy is usually placed in this group although its base is more in philosophy. Yalom (1989), an existential psychotherapist, identifies the four issues which all of us struggle with throughout our lives: death, freedom, existential isolation and meaninglessness.

PERSON-CENTRED COUNSELLING

Person-centred or Client-centred counselling, developed by Carl Rogers in the USA in the 1940s and 1950s, can be seen as the founding work in the humanistic approaches. In *Client Centred Counselling* (1951) Person-centred theory is well known and has been widely taught in the United Kingdom since the 1960s. From the outset, person-centred counselling had a coherent theory and research base. The use of the word 'client' rather than 'patient' conveys one of the fundamental beliefs – that the client is not an object to be treated but a responsible individual to be respected. The unique personal experience of the client is of prime importance as is the counsellor's non-judgemental acceptance of the client.

Rogers stated that six conditions must be in place for change and growth to take place. The two people, counsellor and client, must be in psychological contact; the client must be experiencing vulnerability or anxiety; the counsellor must be genuine or congruent in the relationship; the counsellor must have empathy and unconditional positive regard for the client and communicate this successfully to the client to some degree. In his view, constructive change would follow (Rogers 1957). The theory assumes that given the right conditions the individual will instinctively move and develop to achieve his/her potential. This is described as the actualising tendency.

Person-centred counselling theory has developed since 1957, but Rogers' six conditions are found in most humanistic approaches. Person-centred theory believes that if allowed, human beings will be self-directing, creative, positive and have a sense of self-worth. Adverse experiences knock people off track, leading to low self-worth and low self-esteem, which in turn result in dysfunctional relationships and prevent people from achieving their potential. A client who has been knocked off track can be restored by the right conditions in the counselling relationship. The counsellor facilitates self-discovery and growth through the medium of the authentic relationship with the client. The successful outcome of therapy is increased self-acceptance and a sense of self-worth, a validation of the client as a valuable person worthy of respect. No distinction is made between thoughts, feelings or behaviour. Person-centred counselling is an optimistic theory with an implicit belief of the essential goodness of people.

A child learns and internalises values and beliefs from significant people around him/her and these contribute to the formation of the self-concept. This self-concept may be out of harmony with the ideal self, especially if the individual has learnt to measure him/herself against externally imposed values and behaviour rather than against his/her internal organismic self. The theoretical belief is that the closer the match between self-concept and the ideal self, the better the person will function, with a greater sense of wellbeing and be able to use his/her resources to meet his/her potential. There is no place for the psychoanalytic concepts of the unconscious in person-centred theory; the self is in conscious awareness. However, theorists since Rogers have developed the idea of client material that is at the 'edge of awareness' that can if brought into awareness result in changes to the self-concept. Gendlin developed a four-stage therapeutic model of 'focusing' in order to move such material from the edge to full awareness (Gendlin 1968). This is sometimes described as the 'felt sense'. Such a move into a client's full awareness may lead to changes in the self-concept. A further development has been into relational depth, meaning ' A state of profound contact and engagement between two people, in which each person is fully real with the Other, and able to understand and value the Other's experiences at a high level' (Mearns and Cooper 2005: xii). (This is included in this section although the authors state that the experience of such relational depth is recognised by therapists of all approaches.)

Criticisms of the humanistic approaches

Person-centred counselling is criticised as being unfocused, with no reliable measures of outcomes. If the client sets the goals and assesses their own process how can there ever be reliable outcome measures? The counselling takes as long as it takes – this can be frustrating for clients who want to have some idea of how long it will take to address their problem. Clients can find the emphasis on the 'here and now' unfocused and unhelpful – going nowhere. Person-centred counselling in particular is criticised as ignoring the possibility of human evil, through the belief in the actualising tendency; and this can lead to counsellors finding themselves in conflict with their theoretical approach and ethical codes. The emphasis on acceptance and a lack of boundaries can be taken by the client as the counsellor condoning risky or unethical behaviour.

INTEGRATIVE APPROACHES

Integrative approaches arose from dissatisfaction after finding that a single approach does not work with all clients, or that some clients do not like a particular approach: 'Pure theories and pure techniques are inadequate to explain and treat complex psychological problems: narrow conceptual positions and simplistic answers to major problems are inadequate' (Holmes and Bateman 2002: 4). Roth and Fonagy observe that 'ultimately, theoretical models will have to be integrated, since they are all approximate models of the same phenomenon: the human mind in distress' (2006: 14).

It is common to see both training courses and counsellors and psychotherapists describing themselves as 'integrative'. It is very difficult to know exactly what this means. This section attempts to cover some of the meanings of 'integrative' in counselling theory.

There are several models of integration. Some seek to integrate two or more theoretical approaches and as such do not create a new theoretical approach. Others have developed a process model and fit interventions from various theories into the process. Others use research into the variables which make counselling effective to develop common factors found in all theoretical approaches. It is also possible to make a distinction in integrative approaches between those theories which focus on the relationship and those which focus on specific interventions. The range of integrative approaches is discussed in more detail later in this chapter.

Some of the 'integrative' approaches could also be described as eclectic. The difference between eclectic and integrative was explained by Ian Horton to BACP staff as the difference between a plate of meat and two veg and a plate of stew. With the eclectic meat and two veg, all the elements are separate and you eat them in the combination that suits you best. In the plate of stew the elements have already been integrated for you!

Four forms of integrated approaches are outlined below.

Integration of existing theories to produce a new approach

This may be the combination of two or more approaches to create a new theoretical model and way of working. Cognitive Behavioural Therapy is the clearest and best known example of this; its name clearly indicates the theoretical component parts. The original approaches may also continue unchanged as is the case with cognitive and behavioural therapy. This is one reason for the huge number of theoretical approaches in counselling and psychotherapy. Two more recent examples are Cognitive Analytic Therapy which integrates elements of psychoanalysis and cognitive therapy and Interpersonal Psychotherapy which combines psychodynamic and systemic approaches. These approaches tend to develop their own language to describe theories and also new interventions.

A new theoretical approach is developed based on the process of counselling

This theoretical model is based on the processes of therapy and therapeutic change. Different theoretical approaches are used at different stages of the counselling process. For example, Egan's model focuses on problem management and facilitating client change subdivided into three stages: exploration, understanding and action (1975).

A more recent example would be Clarkson's Relational model (2003). In Clarkson's theory the emphasis is on the therapeutic relationship and the changes in the nature of the relationship between client and counsellor at different stages of counselling. Each form of relationship employs a different theoretical approach. Clarkson's theoretical relationship forms are: the working alliance which establishes and maintains the psychological contact between counsellor and client; the transference/counter-transference relationship which works with the way in which the past experiences of both counsellor and client distort the way they see and relate to each other; the reparative and developmental relationship through which counselling provides what was missing for the client from earlier formative relationships; the person-to-person or real relationship in which the counsellor is authentic and present in the relationship and enables the client to move in this direction and create an open and honest relationship and process; and the transpersonal which links to the spiritual elements of counselling.

'The Common Factors' approach

This approach has its origins in research into the effectiveness of specific theoretical approaches. When research studies into effectiveness were analysed together, that is a meta-analysis, it was discovered that all were more or less similarly effective. This led to the identification of generic features that contributed to good client outcomes, whatever the theoretical approach, that is, the 'common factors' or 'non-specific variables' (that is, variables unconnected to a particular theoretical approach). Common factors are those which were found not only to be consistently present, but which also have a significant positive impact on client outcomes (Wampold 2001).

The common factors which have been identified are: the counsellor's skill in providing empathic understanding, mutually agreed goals and tasks (between counsellor and client), the client's engagement in the counselling, the creation of hope and the client's capacity to form a strong relationship with the counsellor. In particular the relationship between client and counsellor seems to be strongly correlated with the outcome of the counselling (*Psychotherapy Research* 2005). There is evidence to suggest that common factors and factors external to both counsellor and client make a greater contribution to therapeutic change than the specific approach used.

The common factors integrative theoretical approach can be further subdivided into an approach which seeks to use the common factors to develop a single theoretical model which will be effective for all clients and all counsellors. The second approach recognises that there is no 'one true theory'. The common factors should be present in all approaches, but no more than that, and the wide diversity of theories should be welcomed. If clients are encouraged to make meaning of their life and experience that speaks to them, why should this not also apply to counsellors?

Individual integration

A final form of theoretical integration is that which many individual counsellors develop during their working lives (Orlinsky and Ronnestad 2005; Orlinsky et al. 1999; Skovholt and Ronnestad 1992). Some UK-based research (Hollanders and McLeod 1999) found that although many therapists identified with a main theoretical approach, this was used as a base and other theories were integrated into the clinical work.

There are two types of individual integration. The first refers to the mature practice of experienced counsellors which research shows is the normal development (Skovholt and Ronnestad 1992). Although counsellors would still identify themselves with the theoretical approach of their training, their practice in fact integrated elements from other approaches. Irvin Yalom, an existential psychotherapist wrote that 'the therapist must strive to create a new therapy for each patient' (2002: 34). Therapists developed an approach that reflected their own being and which over the years they had learnt worked for clients. As Roth and Fonagy recognise, 'In everyday clinical practice, there is much that is "borrowed" from different orientations by all practitioners' (2006: 15).

Criticisms of integrative approaches

The main criticism of integrative approaches is that of lack of depth. No single theory is studied in enough depth for a counsellor to be able to use it fully, effectively or even safely. This may put the client at risk because the counsellor lacks in-depth knowledge to be aware of contra-indications for that particular approach. This restricts the work to the superficial. Integrative approaches cover over the differences in theories to the detriment of the client and the whole field, as it denies the richness of the diversity. Counsellors wedded to a single theoretical approach can see integrative theories as an attack on the validity of their own model and way of working.

DIFFERENCES IN THEORETICAL APPROACHES AND HOW TO CHOOSE

Some of the differences between the various theoretical approaches will have become clear in this chapter. There are different views of human nature and how we come to be as we are. Some approaches are based on technical interventions, work with specific conditions and have overt goals of symptom reduction or behaviour change. Others see the client as a whole person in a context and the theories are embodied in the relationship between counsellor and client. Some see human beings as in a perpetual state of internal unconscious conflict, riven by primitive urges which we fear to own. Others see human beings as positive growth seeking individuals in need of reparative relationships to get back on track.

The nature of the counsellor–client relationship differs greatly. In CBT there is recognition that a good working relationship contributes to good client outcomes, but this is a working task-focused relationship. The psychodynamic, person-centred and integrative approaches see the therapeutic relationship as the heart of the therapy and the crucible within which change happens. However, the actual way of working is very different. The psychodynamic counsellor will offer interpretations of the transference material of the client and will try to avoid influencing this in any way. The person-centred and humanistic counsellor will actively work to build a genuine real relationship with the client, at times perhaps using some self-disclosure. An integrative counsellor might work in any or all of these ways, depending on the theoretical approach being used.

Another difference in theoretical approaches is the implicit role of the client in the relationship. CBT and some of the related approaches require the active participation of clients both in and between sessions. Some of the other approaches are not surprised by resistance and hostility to counselling and the counsellor at certain stages. The focus of the work varies – from bringing the unconscious into awareness in psychodynamic/psychoanalytic work, to the identification and reduction of symptoms in CBT. Some like CBT have a clear focus, with others it is more implicit and it is the journey not the destination that matters.

Single approach or integrative?

It has already been stated that for students and counsellors at the start of practice, it can be difficult to make use of theory in the session with a client. Theory is useful when reflecting on the session and writing case notes, in case discussions and in supervision. It provides a common language and concepts to debate and discuss. An integrative approach can provide a flexibility which in turn gives more confidence in being able to work with a range of clients and their problems. Some integrative approaches can cause confusion, because if they are not coherent and consistent, it is easy to flounder and have no idea what you are doing or why. In the USA where all training is postgraduate, counsellors train in a range of approaches, what we would describe as eclectic, and then special-ise in a particular approach at doctoral level.

If you choose to study a single theoretical approach, try to keep an open mind and compare what you are learning to other theories. It is easy for training to become more like entry into a religious movement, than train-ing for a professional career.

CONCLUSION

This chapter has given a very brief overview of the main theoretical approaches with the intention of providing enough to guide the choice of approach for anyone considering entering training. No theoretical approach will work well with all clients all of the time. Many counsellors tend to stay with the approach they first train in, or say they do. There is evidence that in fact, counsellors assimilate and adapt their work through experience to produce practice unique to the individual counsellor (Skovholt and Ronnestad 1992).

FURTHER READING

Dryden, W. and A. Reeves (Eds) (2014). *The Handbook of Individual Therapy* (6th edition). London, Sage.
Lister-Ford, C. (Ed.) (2007). *A Short Introduction to Psychotherapy. Short Introductions to the Therapy Professions*. London, Sage.
McLeod, J. (2009). *An Introduction to Counselling*. Maidenhead, McGrawHill/Open University Press.

REFERENCES

Beck, A. T. (1976). *Cognitive Therapy and Emotional Disorders*. New York, International Universities Press.
Bowlby, J. (1979). *The Making and Breaking of Affectional Bonds*. London, Tavistock.
Brown, L. (2010). *Feminist Therapy*. Washington, American Psychological Association.

Casement, A. (2007). 'Psychodynamic Therapy: The Jungian Approach'. In W. Dryden, *Dryden's Handboook of Individual Therapy*. London, Sage.

Clarkson, P. (2003). *The Therapeutic Relationship*. New York, John Wiley & Sons.

Cooper, M. (2008). *Essential Research Findings in Counselling and Psychotherapy*. London, SAGE and BACP.

Cooper, M. and J. McLeod (2011). *Pluralistic Counselling and Psychotherapy*. London, Sage.

de Swaan, A. (1990). *Critical Essays in Health and Welfare*. London, Routledge.

Drisko, J. W. (2004). 'Common factors in psychotherapy outcome: Meta-analytic findings and their implications for practice and research'. *Families in Society* 85(1): 81–90.

Egan, G. (1975). *The Skilled Helper: A Model for Systematic Helping and Interpersonal Relating*. Monterey, CA, Brooks/Cole.

Ellis, A. (1994). *Reason and Emotion in Psychotherapy*. New York, Birch Lane Press.

Eysenck, H. J. (1952). 'The effects of psychotherapy: an evaluation'. *Journal of Consulting Psychology* 16(5): 310–24.

Gendlin, E. T. (1968). 'A theory of personality change'. In. P. Worchel and D. Byrne, *Personality Change*. New York, John Wiley and Sons.

Hollanders, H. and J. McLeod (1999). 'Theoretical orientation and reported practice: a survey of eclecticism among counsellors in Britain'. *British Journal of Guidance and Counselling* 27(3): 405–14.

Holmes, J. and A. Bateman (Eds) (2002). *Integration in Psychotherapy*. Oxford, Oxford University Press.

Maddox, B. (2006). *Freud's Wizard: The Enigma of Ernest Jones*. London, John Murray.

Masson, J. (1990). *Against Therapy*. London, Harper-Collins.

McLeod, J. (2009). *An Introduction to Counselling*. Maidenhead, McGrawHill Open University Press.

Mearns, D. and M. Cooper (2005). *Working at Relational Depth in Counselling and Psychotherapy*. London, Sage.

Orlinsky, D. E. and M. H. Ronnestad (Eds) (2005). *How Psychotherapists Develop: A Study of Therapeutic Work and Professional Growth*. Washington D.C., American Psychology Association.

Orlinsky, D. E., M. Ronnestad, et al. (1999). 'Development of psycho-therapists: concepts, questions, and methods of a collaborative international study'. *Psychotherapy Research* 9(2): 127–53.

Psychotherapy Research (2005). 'Special Issue: The Therapeutic Relationship'. *Psychotherapy Research* 15(1–2).

Rogers, C. R. (1951). *Client Centred Counselling*. Boston, Houghton Mifflin.

Rogers, C. R. (1957). 'The necessary and sufficient conditions of therapeutic personality change.' *Journal of Counselling Psychology* **21**: 95–103.

Rosen, C. C. H. (2012). *A Problem-based Approach to Teaching Employability and Independent Learning Skills*. HEA STEM First annual conference, London.

Roth, A. and P. Fonagy (2006). *What Works for Whom? A Critical Review of Psychotherapy Research* (2nd edition). New York, The Guilford Press.

Sedgwick, D. (1994). *The Wounded Healer: Countertransference from a Jungian Perspective*. London, Routledge.

Skovholt, T. and M. H. Ronnestad (1995). *The Evolving Professional Self: Stages and Themes in Therapist and Counsellor Development*. Chichester, John Wiley and Sons.

Smail, D. (2001). *The Nature of Unhappiness*. London, Robinson.

Topolinski, S. and G. Hertel (2007). 'The role of personality in psychotherapists' careers: Relationship between personality traits, therapeutic schools and job satisfaction.' *Psychotherapy Research* **17**(3): 365–75.

Varlami, E. and R. Bayne (2007). 'Psychological types and counselling psychology trainees' choice of counselling orientation.' *Counselling Psychology Quarterly* **20**(4): 361–73.

Wampold, B. E. (2001). *The Great Psychotherapy Debate: Models, Methods and Findings*. Mahwah, NJ, Erlbaum.

Yalom, I. (1989). *Love's Executioner and Other Tales of Psychotherapy*. New York, Basic Books.

Yalom, I. (2002). *The Gift of Therapy*. London, Piatkus.

5 PERSONAL DEVELOPMENT AND SURVIVING AS A COUNSELLOR

INTRODUCTION

The focus of this chapter is on the personal development of the counsellor. 'Personal therapy' is the phrase used to describe the counselling students may be required to undertake during training. Because this is the generally understood term, it is also used in this chapter. The phrase is used as if it somehow differs from the counselling that the students will deliver to clients. The arguments for and against obligatory personal therapy during training are presented. Suggestions are made on what to look for in a therapist and how to get the best from personal therapy during training. The second section considers some of the pitfalls and survival techniques for newly qualified counsellors. In a profession such as counselling, in which the counsellor's relational skills are the core of the occupation, every practitioner has an ethical obligation for self-care in order to be able to work effectively and ethically. Throughout are pointers to what motivates people to become counsellors.

Everyone who trains to become a counsellor will change during the process and this change and development continues through the professional career. Counsellors may believe that they work to assist clients to change aspects of their understanding or relationships. There is no doubt that counsellors too are changed by the relationships and work with clients (Yalom 2002; Skovholt and Trotter-Mathison 2011).

In order to survive and to work effectively, with the necessary level of empathy and connection, to deliver what Skovholt and Trotter-Mathison call 'consistent emotional caring' (2011: 166), the counsellor needs to build and maintain a balance between care for clients and care for self. If the counsellor cannot care for and support him/herself, then she cannot be fully available to the client. The intensity needed to work effectively in each relationship can lead to burn out. It is easy in the focus on caring for clients to forget about the giver of that care. It is also easy to forget that family and friends make demands for care.

WHERE DO COUNSELLORS COME FROM? WHAT MOTIVATES SOMEONE TO BECOME A COUNSELLOR?

BACP surveys of members indicate that many people come into counselling as a second career, often from professions such as social work, teaching, nursing, careers advice and guidance (BACP 2009). That is, in their careers, many people have already made a commitment to caring for others, and counsellor training is a further development of this. Some people decide to enter training after a positive experience of being a client. Others do an introductory counselling skills course out of interest and find they wish to pursue this to full professional training. Some people have experience of volunteering with an agency like the Samaritans and wish to move from this to a more full-time occupation as a counsellor.

Have you been long in the making?

There is a view that most people have within them the attributes of a counsellor and that becoming a counsellor is a development process. McLeod lists these attributes as interpersonal skills, technical skills, acceptance of others, a good memory, an ability to assess and make sense of someone's story, an ability to understand the wider social context and finally an openness to learning (2009). What is not known is why some people choose to develop those attributes through training and some do not.

It is unnerving to read that your health and physique are influenced by the conditions in which your grandmother lived when she was pregnant with your mother.[1] It is similarly unsettling to learn that the history and dynamics of family relationships may predispose you to become a counsellor and influence how you do the job (Bachelor and Horvath 1999; Rizq and Target 2008, 2010).

Some counsellors therefore, may be predisposed towards entering a caring profession by previous experiences and especially those in early childhood. Most of us have a mix of motives, some deep-seated, even unconscious, others will be more practical. What seems important is that we become aware of these motives and how they may impact upon the work and personal development.

For some people, counselling acts as an unrecognised way to meet their needs, for example to be appreciated or to offset loneliness; perhaps as a form of reparation for what was missing in early family relationships. Some people are motivated by a desire to help other people, others by the need to be appreciated and hope to get that from clients. The perceived rewards may be the motivation; being seen as a counsellor may give some people a sense of identity and social status. Some people may find that

---

[1]The economic conditions during which your grandmother was pregnant with your mother influence you, as your mother as a foetus already had all the eggs in her ovaries, one of which, when mature and fertilised, became you.

they are always the person turned to by friends and family to be a listening ear and want to develop these skills and attributes. The idea of being able to help others in distress can be very seductive and may offer a form of voyeurism into the complex and at time dramatic lives of clients.

A further issue that counsellors need to address is that of the personal reward they get from being a counsellor. It is necessary and legitimate that as counsellors, we have some of our personal needs met through the work. This is not unique to counselling. It is part of what motivates people to go to work every day. Work can offer many different rewards, companionship, intellectual stimulation, money to pay the bills, an avoidance of boredom and a sense of achievement.

Below are examples of three counsellors and their explanations of their motivations to become counsellors:

> One counsellor had experience of mental illness in the family from an early age and wanted to understand more about this and how to help people with similar problems.

> A careers adviser came to think that there must be more that could be done to help the young people she worked with.

> Another counsellor began as a Samaritan and when family commitments allowed, undertook counsellor training out of interest, never expecting it to lead to a new career.

Activity

Look at your family and life before starting training. How many of the factors given apply to you? Add any other motivations you can think of. Then rank them all in order of importance to you.

Table 5.1 *Good and bad motivations for becoming a counsellor*

Motivating factor	Self-assessment
Desire to help others	
Intellectual stimulation	
Own emotional growth	
Prestige and status	
Curiosity about people	
Unresolved personal needs	
Desire to feel powerful	
Unresolved emotional distress	
Living through clients' lives	

Source: Aveline (2007: 521–2)

WHAT HAPPENS TO PEOPLE DURING TRAINING?

This section covers some of the issues and processes that can happen early in a counsellor's development, both in training and the early years of practice. Training presents students with a set of skills, knowledge and ways to do things, with the implication that these are the 'right' ways. It is important for the student to get these right in order to qualify. 'Humour may take a holiday during training' (Skovholt and Trotter-Mathison 2011: 40–1).

During training and in the early years of practice, counsellors can find themselves behaving in ways that are described here; for example taking on one or more of the following roles: imposter, messiah and wounded healer.

The sense of being an imposter is common especially in training. In my training group, many of us were struck with our arrogance that we thought we could help other people, when we felt much more in need of help than any potential client. Part of this came from our shared anxiety about impending placements. We feared the sort of clients we might get and what we were expected to 'do with them'! Another contributor to the anxiety was our growing understanding of the complexity of human distress and mental illness and how little we knew.

The 'messiah' role, can also act as a protection against anxiety and fear. The messiah counsellor presents as a knowledgeable powerful loving therapist. This rather grandiose professional self can be reinforced by some clients who idealise anyone helping them. Some counsellors may find it easier to give help than ask for it. Such counsellors may find people unwilling or unable to give help when it is requested if they have established themselves as such a powerful 'messiah'.

The 'wounded healer' is a term found in the literature with a range of meanings. The wounded healer paradigm holds that within every healer is a wound that may influence the choice of occupation and also contributes to the effectiveness of the therapist. One sense of this is that every person is 'wounded' in some way. The wounded healer uses their own experience and the compassion derived from it as a source to heal others. A more negative position is one where the 'healer' uses clients to heal their own 'wounds', which can lead to abusive relationships with clients. One interviewee who had just finished a Counselling Skills course, thought that many on the course fitted into this category. They were impatient to start 'healing' clients!

Personal therapy

There are several aspects to the issue of personal therapy for counsellors. The first is the issue of mandatory personal therapy during training, the second is the differences between theoretical approaches on the issue of personal therapy, and the third is personal therapy after training.

Personal therapy has been described as 'the symbolic core of professional identity in the mental health field' (Henry, Sims and Spray 1974, quoted in Geller, Norcross et al. 2005: 3). The phrase carries with it a sense of mysticism. If I had spent thousands of pounds on three- or five-times-a-week training analysis for several years, I would probably take this view. If on the other hand I had barely engaged in my course's required 20 hours of therapy, spending the sessions mentally rating the counsellor's performance in terms of empathy, skills and application of theory, my view might be different.

Mandatory personal therapy during training

The place of personal therapy during training has been the subject of much debate (Chaturvedi 2013). In Europe and the UK this 'personal therapy' is often an obligatory requirement of counselling and psychotherapy training courses. Such a requirement is found only in the psychological therapies and not in all. Psychiatrists are not required to have had a psychiatric illness in order to qualify. When personal analysis was introduced as a requirement for psychoanalytic training Freud did not partake (Feltham 2013).

Arguments in favour of personal therapy during training   The rationale for therapy during training can be divided into the personal and the professional, underpinned by a belief that undertaking therapy will have positive outcomes in both areas. One argument in favour of therapy is the need to know oneself. In counselling 'one's personal life is a central component of professional functioning' (Skovholt and Trotter-Mathison 2011: 48). An understanding of self and self-awareness are therefore key values in counselling and counselling is a common method used to develop this self-knowledge and with it an increased personal maturity or 'soundness'.

Each of us has a unique view of the world, with its unique quirks and distortions. These do not usually matter much in everyday life, indeed we are unaware of them or the impact they may have most of the time. However, in a therapeutic relationship, such distortions can have a profound impact.

The heart of counselling is the relationship between counsellor and client, often described as the therapeutic alliance. In order to be able to build and maintain this relationship a counsellor must be able to reflect upon him/herself and seek understanding and insight into themselves in order to be able to be fully present with the client and to be able to separate self from client in the work. The essential capability required is that of self-reflection. This is both the ability to and the habit of reflecting on one's own life and experiences in an open and critical way. The effect of varying levels of a counsellor's reflexive ability is discussed later in this chapter (and see also Chapter 7 for the relationship between reflexivity and research). Therapy during training represents one of the ways in which students can begin to identify their unique view of the world and the impact this may have on responses to clients. However, it is possible that the student who has had a positive experience of their own therapy may inadvertently generalise their unique experience into work with clients.

Another argument for personal therapy as an essential requirement is that it can be dangerous to work as a therapist without it: a 'therapist can only go as far with the patient as she can go herself' (Aveline 2007). This is the position taken by many people with a psychodynamic approach. The argument for this, relates to the motivations which bring people into training. There is a belief that would-be counsellors are motivated by their own unresolved issues and unmet needs. Engaging in therapy during training enables the counsellor to identify these and address them, or at least become aware of them and how such issues might impact on work with clients.

A further argument in favour of personal therapy during training is that it seems to be a powerful socialisation experience for students, and act as an initiation rite into the profession.

Personal therapy ties the student to the discipline in a more powerful way than the other elements of training; especially if the therapeutic relationship and the outcomes are positive. The student is living proof that counselling works, and has been both an active participant in a transformational process and recipient and observer of the delivery of effective counselling. The personal therapy validates the student as 'fit' for the role of counsellor and in particular the theoretical approach in which they are training (Grimmer 2005).

Arguments against personal therapy during training   A powerful argument against obligatory therapy during training is the coercive nature of such a requirement and the possible lack of choice of therapist. In the 'real' world clients decide when they want to engage in counselling and have an internal reason for so doing. Students do it because they have to, in order to pass the course. These factors are believed to undermine any possible positive outcomes. Certainly I used to try to avoid taking on counselling students who had to have a set number of hours of therapy because I disliked the prescribed number of hours and with some students doubted the commitment to the process. Students can find it difficult to fully engage as clients. As one said, 'It was difficult, I think I did. But I was aware of seeing how she was doing it.'

There is some evidence to suggest that therapy during training can lead to the trainee becoming caught up in their personal issues at the expense of both client and course work. There can be a negative impact on the work with clients (Macaskill 1992). In some institutions there can be boundary blurring, where the therapist also has a teaching role. Personal therapy can also cause negative emotional and financial stress to trainees. It has been argued that the financial costs in addition to course fees exclude people from training on the grounds of affordability rather than ability and as a result restrict the social diversity in counselling. Macaskill, who researched the effects of therapy in training, questioned whether undertaking one's own therapy was the best way to gain the skills and qualities needed to be an effective therapist (1988). There are other ways to achieve self-awareness (Johns 2009; Bolton 2010; McLeod 2009).

THEORETICAL APPROACHES AND PERSONAL THERAPY

For many theoretical approaches, personal therapy is the only valid means of achieving self-awareness. For other approaches a wider range of activities can be undertaken to achieve the same end such as personal development groups, and reflective journals. Psychodynamic courses may place more emphasis on and require more hours of personal therapy. The psychodynamic view is that personal therapy is the only way to gain sufficient self-awareness to be able to recognise and work with transference and counter-transference. One psychodynamic course requires students to undertake a minimum of one hour a week during the four-year training course. Humanistic and person-centred trainings often take the view that such self-knowledge can be gained through a wider range of activities. For example, one humanistic course requires students to have eight hours of personal therapy a year during a two-year course and attend a weekly experiential group. Some person-centred courses see the dynamics of the training group as means of gaining self-awareness. Family therapy and cognitive behavioural courses usually do not make personal therapy a mandatory training requirement. These varying beliefs appear to be 'articles of faith' and as such not open to debate. However, all approaches support students entering personal therapy to work on issues that may arise during training.

At times, the issue of personal therapy has been used to support claims to superiority of one theoretical approach over another. The British Association for Counselling's accreditation criteria became one battle ground in the 1990s between the psychodynamic and person-centred approaches. The outcome was a compromise which required applicants to have had 40 hours of therapy or an equivalent activity consistent with the core theoretic model of the training.

WHAT SHOULD A STUDENT LOOK FOR IN A COUNSELLOR?

Evidence suggests that counselling is more likely to have a good result if there is a good match between counsellor and client, and that a positive relationship develops in the first three to five sessions. The elements in a good match are shared role expectations, compatible styles, congruence and reciprocity in expectations, styles and philosophy. More contentious may be the finding that a convergence of social and cultural values may lead to better outcomes as do reciprocal personality dynamics (Geller, Norcross et al. 2005).

My 'perfect' counsellor will be deeply human, not a cold professional, she will show me warmth, respect, even liking. She will listen and understand what I am trying to communicate, but won't assume that she understands without checking. She will work at my pace and will not force her own interpretations or judgements on me. I don't want a 'nodding dog' of clichéd phrases and encouraging murmurs all the time. I want her to make it safe enough for me to go to places that might be disturbing or distressing, and for her to encourage me to do so. I would like my counsellor to laugh and cry with me at times. I want to feel confident that she knows what we are doing. It may be clear to some readers that as I write this, I have a real counsellor in mind.

WHAT TO FOCUS ON IN THERAPY DURING TRAINING

This section aims to help students get the most out of any obligatory therapy requirement, recognising that some people will have a negative reaction to being told to go and get counselling now and for this long. If the training course requires students to undertake a set number of sessions, then it is sensible to get the most out of the sessions. Below are some of the ways to do this.

If your initial reaction was one of opposition and resistance, it is worth taking time to reflect on this. Is this part of how you respond to being told to do anything? Or is it related to being asked to 'expose' yourself to a stranger? If the latter – then it might be helpful to link this to how clients may feel. Perhaps there is a fear that you will reveal yourself as totally unsuited to becoming a counsellor. If so, you will not be alone in this. An exploration of motivation and how the training is affecting you are very important and helpful areas to look at. It matters to remember that the counsellor is there for you. He/she is on your side. It may be helpful to discuss any misgivings and uncertainties with fellow students and the counsellor. It is useful to keep such notes and refer back to them when you have a reluctant client in the future.

Personal therapy during training will be a first experience for some students but not for others. Students who have had counselling before will almost certainly compare the experiences, but the situation and reasons for entering therapy are different. Therapy 'virgins' obviously will not be able to make such a comparison. All students will be able to use the experience for reflection on their own practice as well as the personal gains.

Possible areas to explore in counselling during training

It is often difficult for students to know where to begin or what to focus on, as they are not necessarily entering counselling as a result of a private need or a powerful sense that something needs to change.

An obvious area to explore would be the motivations for entering the profession. As mentioned earlier in the chapter, research suggests that counsellors may have some elements in their histories that predispose them to counselling, for example, loneliness and outsider status in childhood (Bachelor and Horvath 1999; Rizq and Target 2008, 2010; Skovholt and Trotter-Mathison 2011). The quality of childhood attachment and losses has been found to correlate to the effectiveness of professional attachment (Bachelor and Horvath 1999; Rizq and Target 2008, 2010). A recent study found that the majority of therapists in the cohort had insecure attachments (Rizq and Target 2008, 2010). This supports the idea that some people who enter the talking therapies as a profession have had a childhood in which they were required to meet the narcissistic needs of parents, and this has led to the development of a false sense of self, of being someone who meets the needs of others and hence to counselling as a profession.

Exploring one's own attachment style could be a productive area of work that might enable the counsellor to become aware of areas of risk and address these in therapy. Research suggests that different attachment patterns are likely to influence how people work as therapists (Bachelor and Horvath 1999). For example, a counsellor whose past relationships have led them to be self-critical may be more likely to be subtly hostile to clients replaying earlier relationship patterns of insecure attachment and may invite similar responses from clients. There is evidence to suggest that therapists with secure attachment work differently to therapists without secure attachments. The former seem better able to form an early therapeutic alliance, the latter tend to intervene at greater depth (Bachelor and Horvath 1999; Rizq and Target 2008, 2010).

Exploration of motivation and attachment styles may lead into expectations of the work as a counsellor. It may be productive to consider the theoretical approach chosen as there is some tentative evidence to suggest that certain Myers-Briggs personality types fit better with some theoretical approaches than others (Varlami and Bayne 2007).

Counsellors need to be able to deal with strong emotions without being overwhelmed and personal therapy can be a great help in recognising existing coping mechanisms and reviewing the appropriateness of these for use in counselling. The increased self-awareness will help the counsellor hold and share the client's strong emotions of fear, anger and despair, rather than deny them or take them in. In early practice it is not unusual for a client to skip out of the session leaving the novice counsellor groaning under the weight that seems to have been dropped on their shoulders. Being a trainee in therapy does provide the student with the chance to observe an experienced counsellor at work. But this should be something to be gained during reflection on the therapy, not consciously done during sessions. A student doing this during therapy is probably using it as a barrier to avoid engaging in the work, by remaining in an observer role. It is useful and important to reflect on what aspects of the process worked for you and which did not. But, when in practice it is important not to assume that what worked for you will work for a client presenting with a similar issue.

WHAT TO DO IF THE RELATIONSHIP BETWEEN THE STUDENT AND THE COUNSELLOR IS NOT WORKING?

This is a tricky issue, if the counsellor has any influence on the outcome of the training, in other words, if the student has to 'pass' the therapy in some way. The counsellor should negotiate a contract with the student, for the number and cost of sessions, the boundaries of confidentiality, which will include any assessment of the student. Such assessment is unlikely, but circumstances could arise in which the therapist was legally obliged to break confidentiality (see Chapter 6 on Ethics).

The relationship is one of the main areas where things can go wrong. The relationship may feel punitive rather than empathic. The counsellor may make negative, critical interventions, or appear not to understand. She may impose a direction on the work opposite to what the student wants. There may seem to be no progress, nothing seems to be happening. If things go wrong, students may feel that they do not have the 'Did Not Attend' (DNA) option open to clients. The options are to either raise the issue or withdraw and just get through the required number of sessions. The best and bravest thing to do is to raise the issue and try to address it openly. Therapeutic relationships can recover from such breakdowns and have positive outcomes. This can also be very positive learning for the student when a similar alliance breakdown happens in practice.

WHAT DO STUDENTS GET FROM THERAPY DURING TRAINING? WHAT ARE THE OUTCOMES OF SUCCESSFUL THERAPY FOR THE STUDENT?

Resistance to obligatory therapy during training is not uncommon. Some students may feel that they have no issues to address, no problems, other than finding the time and money to have the required sessions. Others may know that they have issues and consider training the wrong time and place to open up such painful exploration. Learning is still possible, but of a different nature. The resistant student may be given the chance to observe how an experienced counsellor addresses such resistance, and as a result find him/herself engaging in the process.

One common helpful outcome is personal and professional growth which together can help in the development of reflexivity. A further positive outcome is increased empathy with clients and a sense of humility. Some students will be able to work through conflicts and attachment patterns that would impact on their work with clients if left unresolved. Validation as a counsellor as fit to enter the same profession as one's therapist has already been mentioned. This reinforces the concept of personal therapy as a major part of the socialisation process and symbolic rite of passage. Please do not take this to mean that you cannot be a 'true' counsellor if your training course does not insist on personal therapy.

Conclusions on personal therapy during training

It is very difficult to come to any conclusion about mandatory therapy during training as all the theoretical approaches seem to produce competent and ethical counsellors. Much of the research into the effects of therapy during training has been carried out in the USA, often with groups other than counsellors, such as social workers and psychologists. More recently there has been research in the UK. All the studies have been very small, usually under 20 participants. It is therefore difficult to be confident about making generalisations from these studies. However, there are enough similarities in the findings to include them in this book to stimulate thinking.

The evidence of a positive impact on client work is either negative or inconclusive (Geller, Norcross et al. 2005; Chaturvedi 2013). One of the goals of therapy during training is to improve the clinical effectiveness of the student. It is argued that the more emotionally mature the counsellor is the better the clinical work, by having greater understanding of their own intra- and interpersonal dynamics and therefore of those of other people. This should therefore increase effectiveness and lead to positive client outcomes. However, there is inconclusive evidence that therapists' therapy, whether in training or when in practice, increases effectiveness or enhances client outcomes. As Grimmer (2005) points out, this is something of a paradox. Some theoretical approaches believe that a counsellor should only deliver the intensity of therapy they have experienced themselves, in terms of number of sessions a week.

It may not be possible to prove that having therapy improves client outcomes, but experienced counsellors report overwhelmingly positive outcomes from their perspective (Geller, Norcross et al. 2005). If a positive experience in therapy was the only factor that contributed to positive client outcomes, then it could be argued that every client who had effective therapy or a positive outcome was de facto a trained counsellor!

As McLeod (2009: 625) points out, it is impossible to disaggregate the effect of therapy from the other aspects of training to come to any reliable conclusion. Research shows that the quality of the therapeutic relationship is a good indicator of client outcome regardless of the theoretical approach used (Bachelor and Horvath 1999). It is common sense to think that a good therapeutic experience during training will influence a student's future client work. Despite this lack of evidence, most courses will require students to undertake an amount of personal therapy during training and most students will engage willingly.

ARE THERE DIFFERENCES IN THE THERAPY RECEIVED BY THE 'MAN IN THE STREET' AND A STUDENT?

It appears that there are more similarities than differences. The differences that do exist can be critical to the nature and effectiveness of the therapy. The client has chosen to enter counselling because she does not want something in her life to continue as it is. It may be she wants understanding rather than change, but she is choosing an active form of help. The student is meeting a course requirement, therefore it is not a free choice and there may be no immediate issue or concern that calls for attention. The client may not know very much about counselling in general or the specific approach of the therapist. The student is actively studying the approach and will be curious to see it in action. The therapist may have to make an assessment of the student's suitability to pass the course and enter the profession. Both therapist and student may therefore be judging each other. This is not to say that clients do not also judge their counsellors. Both client and student may be resistant. Quite a few counsellors I know do not enjoy working with students in order for the student 'to tick the box'.

Clients tend to be deferential towards counsellors, leaving the relationship rather than expressing concerns when things seem to be going wrong. Students may feel obliged to stick it out for the required number of sessions, but not engage fully if they are unhappy about the relationship or the focus of the work.

PERSONAL THERAPY DURING PROFESSIONAL CAREER

Research in the USA has shown that an overwhelming majority of therapists enter into counselling during their careers, often more than once. In other words, experienced counsellors, like other professionals, use their profession when they need help (Geller, Norcross et al. 2005; Skovholt and Trotter-Mathison 2011). It is not known if there is a similar level of therapy in the UK. What seems clear is that counsellors do have therapy for themselves after training, to deal with personal issues from everyday life, unresolved conflicts that have been brought to the fore by client material and for support for the work, in addition to supervision. This indicates that practitioners have confidence in what they offer to the public. There is one very important difference between counselling in the USA and the United Kingdom. In the USA counsellors are only required to have supervision until they gain a licence to practise, unlike the UK where supervision is a requirement throughout professional life.

A working counsellor begins, maintains and ends several intense individual relationships every working day, day in day out. These multiple professional attachments cause a high level of 'emotional wear and tear' and in extreme cases can lead to counsellor 'burn out'. Just as you would service a car, counsellors also need to service themselves. 'Oil' and 'brake' checks need particular attention, especially as we are not in a position to get a new model if the old one fails.

Therapy Today carried a column by a counsellor starting in private practice, which gave a vivid account of how it felt –

'Sometimes I feel completely taken over ...'

'I feel overwhelmed, stressed and resentful.'

'You don't know the meaning of the word tired until you become a therapist.'

'Nothing could have prepared me for the strains these new relationships would put on my long-standing ones.!'

The challenge that faces the counsellor is to find a balance between caring for the clients and caring for the self. For women, who form the majority of the counsellors in the UK this can be a particular challenge given the socialisation of women to be the care givers. It is one-sided caring, constant interpersonal sensitivity often with ambiguous outcomes.

EARLY CAREER EXPERIENCES

Everyone in every profession has been new to it, unsure if they are suited to the work, anxious about making mistakes, about being seen as not good enough.

At the start of work as a counsellor every client is an unknown. This of course is true of every client throughout a whole career, but at the start they seem even more unknown. The new counsellor has to try to bring together theory and practice while establishing a therapeutic alliance, without the security of fellow students to talk things through with. It is no wonder that new counsellors are often anxious: 'Being lost and confused in the fog of early practice is a rite of passage' (Skovholt and Trotter-Mathison 2011: 87). These experiences in early practice are universal: 'In time you are no longer afraid of your clients' (Skovholdt and Ronnestad 1992: 96). One reason for this reduction in anxiety is that counsellors learn from each client, a powerful form of professional development that continues throughout practice, especially when connected to good supervision and personal reflection.

One way new counsellors try to address this natural anxiety is to apply what has been learnt in training, but theory does not always correlate with the client's unique presentation and responses: 'I didn't know what I was doing' (Skovholt and Trotter-Mathison 2011: 81). I recall feeling quite confident about the first session, I had been taught and had practised that, even the second and third sessions, but then what did I do if they came back for more? I had yet to learn that the client is an equal partner in the process, and it didn't all rest with me.

It may be tempting to 'blame' the client, and to stick resolutely to the theoretical model, in the same way as students in therapy tend to 'blame' the therapist not the therapeutic model when the relationship is not working well. This may temporarily alleviate the anxiety, but it does not result in learning and development in the counsellor. A better and more difficult response is to reflect on what is happening and talk about it in supervision and with supportive colleagues. Counsellors never come to the end of their professional development; most of us would be bored stiff if we did. The complexity and ambiguity of practice, which is one of the stresses of early practice, later becomes one of its great delights.

The goal of counselling is for the client to find some sort of resolution of whatever is troubling them. Often this is shortened to a goal of client change. If a client does not seem to be finding any sort of resolution or change, the new counsellor can experience this as a negative judgement on his own skills and abilities and wonder if he is not good enough – not empathic enough, making poor interpretations, not caring enough, maybe doing harm to the client.

I recall a student who had just started a placement, coming to group supervision angry and perplexed after seeing a client who had lost a child: 'I did everything right but she still wouldn't cry!'

At the start of practice, it is easy to have unrealistic expectations of one's own power to bring about change in the client, and the rate of change. There is a tendency for new counsellors to gauge their success only by client change, and this can undermine confidence. This anxiety can be both increased and decreased by session-by-session outcome measures. Clients will change (or not) in their own time, not yours. It is better to take in a broader range of feedback such as supervisor and colleagues. If counsellors measure themselves only against client change they will increase their insecurity and fragility and possibly become too insecure and threatened to learn. Counsellors are very tender and fragile when they start practice and need to find ways to gain confidence and strength.

Some clients will not improve with you as their counsellor. Some clients will not improve with anyone. These are hard lessons to accept early in a career. Such clients challenge the belief structure of the talking therapies and of individual counsellors. As a counsellor gains in experience he becomes aware of the types of clients he works well with and the reasons for this. A counsellor working in private practice may be able to be selective over clients. A counsellor working in an agency, will have less choice. It has been my experience that counselling service intake staff are often very skilled at matching clients to counsellors if the diary allows.

One of the findings in research into the factors in effective therapy is that client responses to therapist's behaviour are not consistent. Thus therapist self-disclosure may enhance the quality of some relationships. Transference interpretations may facilitate insight in some clients but be experienced as criticism by others and lead to defensiveness. The conclusion is that counsellors cannot get it right with every client and must be alert to how and when things go wrong in the relationship. In time, counsellors learn humility, that the counsellor is only one element in the process. Paradoxically, such a sense of humility and relative powerlessness can also lead to an enhanced confidence and better counselling.

Counselling is a hard discipline for people who like to know they are doing a good job, as this sort of feedback from clients is rare and we can never know how much we contributed to client outcomes. This is one of the negative aspects of counselling. Counsellors below share some of the negative aspects of the work.

> 'I thought the work was going well, we'd been working together for some time. He seemed to trust me. Then I encouraged him to go a bit deeper. He never came back. I can only trust in the process and believe that I did my best with him.'

> 'The worst thing for me, is having to face up to myself sometimes.'

> 'The endless not knowing. No knowing if the session was any use.'

> 'The isolation, I can't go home and talk about work, say, Oh, I met someone today who ...'

THE ELEMENTS OF SELF-CARE

Counsellors should look after themselves, pay attention to, recognise and meet their own needs and not see this as selfish and therefore bad. Some of the elements that make up this 'self-care' are outlined below.

Boundaries

In training counsellors are taught about the importance of establishing clear boundaries with clients, but there are other internal boundaries to set. It is important to try to ensure that clients do not intrude into personal life – one counsellor talks of dreaming about clients in the first year of practice and how these professional relationships seemed to be taking precedence over existing private and personal ones. It is important to separate the professional from the private and personal.

Some of these are clearly articulated in such documents as the BACP *Ethical Framework for Counsellors and Psychotherapists* (BACP 2013). Emotional boundaries are more difficult to monitor and hold, and it is not unusual to find emotions from client work seeping into private time. This is described by Skovholdt and Trotter-Mathison as a 'porous boundary', as if the counsellor is a piece of kitchen towel soaking up the emotions of the clients and forgetting to throw it in the bin before going home (Skovholt and Trotter-Mathison 2011).

Counsellors have to learn to separate their own needs from the professional relationships they make with clients. The client's task is not to meet the counsellor's emotional needs. It is for this reason that the development of self-awareness is seen as essential for counsellors. Self-awareness will prevent a counsellor falling into the messiah trap of grandiosity, in which it is much easier to help others than seek help for oneself.

Activity

Look carefully at your personal relationships.

- When was the last time you asked for or received help from a friend?
- What was the response?
- When was the last time a friend asked for help from you?
- What was the response?
- What is the balance of giving and taking with your closest friends?

Saying no

It is all too easy to fall into a pattern of never saying no, even to unreasonable requests. This 'hero/heroine' pattern compounds the imbalance between client care and self-care. Counsellors spend their working lives giving attention and emotional energy to other people, putting the needs of others before their own needs. This can include not only clients but family, friends and colleagues. This one-way caring has to be counter balanced, because the counsellor's own wellbeing is essential for professional competence. This focus on self-care can be difficult for female counsellors who are socialised to care for other people. Yet, Skovholt and Trotter-Mathison state unequivocally that 'psychological wellness is an ethical imperative' (2011: 166).

Supervision

Supervision represents another element in self-care. It is the place where the counsellor can express and explore the demands of practice and the relationships with clients (Wheeler and Richards 2007). A place that offers 'safe uncertainty', as well as support and challenge when needed (Starr, Ciclitira et al. 2012).

Self-care

Counsellors need to nurture themselves, feed themselves in whatever way works for them. There is nothing wrong with meeting your own needs. While it may seem natural that counsellors should seek counselling to help deal with the stress of work, and many do, this may not always be helpful. Other non-therapeutic activities can be more helpful. One reason for such a recommendation is that counselling demands intense focus on interpersonal relationships, to use the same medium for support and stress management may be counter-productive, by maintaining a

therapeutic perspective when a complete change is called for. Operating/
responding from a therapeutic perspective can harm personal relationships. Domestic discussions over whose turn it is to put the rubbish out
are usually not helped by a transference interpretation, however valid you
may think it. After settling the rubbish issue, I took up running – other
counsellors have other ways.

Several counsellors I know use groups of supportive colleagues for this.
One group comprises colleagues from within the profession, the other a
very mixed group who meet in the pub on Fridays to put the world to
rights. Another, a trainer of counsellors has belonged to a self-led non-
task oriented group of other counsellors (also known as a T group) for
15 years that meets every two months. Both have been working in counselling for over 20 years.

Counselling is very tiring. To an outsider the counsellor may be sitting
in a room listening to people all day, but like swans, he is paddling furi-
ously under the water, while appearing effortless above the surface. In
addition the counsellor may never know if the work together had a successful outcome. This in itself can be very draining. It is impossible to
know if the client who stops attending does so because the work is done,
or because the counsellor never managed to engage them. 'Losing' a client
for whatever reason, can feel like bereavement and one that cannot be
openly talked about except in supervision because of the confidential
nature of the work. It can trigger the emotional responses of bereavement,
such as anger, grief and hopelessness. Sometimes, a client will commit
suicide, whatever the counsellor does. This has an impact on the family
and friends and also on the counsellor. Losing a client in this way early in
a career can do great damage to a counsellor's developing confidence.

THE JOYS OF COUNSELLING

The stress mentioned above is more than compensated for by a client's
'aha! moment'. Two examples stand out for me: One, the words from a client: 'I hadn't seen it like that before.' The other was seeing a shy anxious
client walking upright and making eye contact in the University coffee bar.
This was as powerful a form of feedback as any words.

Below counsellors share some of the best things about counselling.

> 'The privilege of hearing different stories. Clients enrich my understanding of
> myself and the world.'

> 'I just find it fascinating. I enjoy the one-to-one in-depth talking.'

> 'I want to make a difference.'

'Having those conversations when you are both way below the surface, and both still breathing. Pulling things together.'

'Always finding something unexpected and being part of the process.'

CONCLUSION

How do we know if we are good enough?

We have come through the messiah trap and the imposter syndrome and recognised and set in place some support and nurturing for ourselves. Then how do we know if we are doing a good enough job? It is almost impossible to define 'good enough' for in some cases this will depend on the context in which the counsellor works and who is assessing 'good enough'. For example, in IAPT (Improving Access to Psychological Therapies) services a certain reduction in scores on routine assessment instruments such as the Generalised Anxiety Disorder Assessment (GAD 7) and the Patient Health Questionnaire (PHQ9) will be the measure of good enough for all therapists in the service. In some EAPs (Employee Assistance Programmes) good enough will be judged on client feedback forms. For the individual counsellor, good enough can mean knowing that he was fully present and engaged with the client, whatever the outcome.

Two aspects are essential in seeking an answer to this question. One is self-reflection on the work with each client, and the second is supportive feedback from supervisor and colleagues. Good supervision is a constant support, mentoring and learning throughout professional practice. Supervision holds the new counsellor and provides a safe place to explore. What counsellors learn from this triangulation of feedback over time is that each counsellor will be better with some clients than others, and some clients will engage in the process, others will not. Some will be a joy to work with, others will flood the counsellor with negative emotions and blame for their problems. Counsellors will have to work with all of this.

The characteristics the counsellor takes into the counselling room will interact with those of the client and both will influence the nature of the therapeutic relationship: 'the therapeutic relationship itself can represent a therapeutic intervention' (Bachelor and Horvath 1999: 161). Counsellors are in an occupation that has an ethical requirement for continued learning, development and self-reflection. They have the privilege of sharing with strangers journeys of discovery. If you don't like dealing with the unknown, counselling is not the job for you.

REFERENCES

Aveline, M. (2007). 'The training and supervision of individual therapists'. In W. Dryden (Ed.), *Dryden's Handbook of Individual Therapy*. London, Sage: 515–48.

Bachelor, A. and A. Horvath (1999). 'The therapeutic relationship'. In M. A. Hubble, B. L. Duncan and S. D. Miller (Eds), *The Heart and Soul of Change: What Works in Therapy*. Washington, DC, American Psychological Society: 133–78.

BACP (2013). *Ethical Framework for Good Practice in Counselling and Psychotherapy*. Lutterworth, BACP.

BACP. (2009). Membership Survey. Lutterworth, BACP.

Bolton, G. (2010). *Reflective Practice: Writing and Professional Development*. London, Sage.

Chaturvedi, S. (2013). 'Mandatory personal therapy: does the evidence justify the practice? In debate.' *British Journal of Guidance and Counselling* **41**(4): 454–60.

Feltham, C. (2013). *Counselling and Counselling Psychology. A Critical Examination*. Ross-on-Wye, PCCS Books.

Geller, J. D., J. C. Norcross, et al. (Eds) (2005). *The Psychotherapist's Own Psychotherapy. Patient and Clinician Perspectives*. New York, Oxford University Press.

Grimmer, A. (2005). 'Personal Therapy: researching a knotty problem.' *Therapy Today* **16**(7): 37–40.

Johns, C. (2009). *Becoming a Reflective Practitioner*. Chichester, Wiley-Blackwell.

Macaskill, N. (1988). 'Personal therapy as a training requirement: the lack of supporting evidence.' In C. Feltham (Ed.), *Controversies in Psychotherapy and Counselling*. London, Sage.

Macaskill, N. (1992). 'Personal therapy in the training of psychotherapists: Is it effective?' *British Journal of Psychotherapy* **4**(3): 219–26.

McLeod, J. (2009). *An Introduction to Counselling*. Maidenhead, Open University Press.

Rizq, R. and M. Target (2008). 'The power of being seen: an interpretive phenomenological analysis of how experienced counselling psychologists describe the meaning and significance of personal therapy in clinical practice.' *British Journal of Guidance and Counselling* **36**(2): 131–53.

Rizq, R. and M. Target (2010). '"If that's what I need, it could be what someone else needs." Exploring the role of attachment and reflective function in counselling psychologists' accounts of how they use personal therapy in clinical practice: a mixed methods study.' *British Journal of Guidance and Counselling* **38**(4): 459–81.

Skovholt, T. M. and M. H. Ronnestad (1992). *The Evolving Professional Self: Stages and Themes in Therapist and Counselor Development.* Wiley Series in Psychotherapy. New York, John Wiley.

Skovholt, T.M. and M. Trotter-Mathison (2011). *The Resilient Practitioner. Burnout Prevention and Self-care Strategies for Counselors, Therapists and Health Professionals.* New York, London, Routledge Taylor and Francis Group.

Starr, F., K. Ciclitira, et al. (2012). 'Comfort and Challenge: a thematic analysis of female clinicians' experiences of supervision.' *Psychology and Psychotherapy* DOI: 10.1111/j.2044-8341.2012.02063.x.

Varlami, E. and R. Bayne (2007). 'Psychological types and counselling psychology trainees' choice of counselling orientation.' *Counselling Psychology Quarterly* **20**(4): 361–73.

Wheeler, S. and K. Richards (2007). *The Impact of Clinical Supervision on Counsellors and Therapists, Their Practice and Their Clients. A Systematic Review of the Literature.* Lutterworth, BACP.

Yalom, I. (2002). *The Gift of Therapy.* London, Piatkus.

6   ETHICS IN COUNSELLING

INTRODUCTION

This chapter considers the nature and cultural context of ethics and the place of ethics in counselling. It presents the use and practical application of ethics in common aspects of counselling work. The main features of the BACP *Ethical Framework for Good Practice in Counselling and Psychotherapy* are outlined and the demands the Framework places on counsellors (BACP 2010). Finally it considers what goes wrong in counselling, how complaints arise and are addressed, using information derived from the operation of the BACP Professional Conduct Process. The most important point this chapter makes is that counsellors need something practical to use when making difficult moral judgements and decisions.

At first glance ethics looks simple. Readers might assume that counsellors behave ethically. It is more accurate to recognise that not all counsellors behave ethically all the time.

DEFINITION OF ETHICS AND USES OF ETHICS

Dictionaries define ethics as either a system of moral principles which are used to govern the behaviour of both individuals and groups, such as professions, or as the assessment of the moral fitness of a decision or action. Definitions also include moral values around human behaviour. Therefore to behave ethically is to act in keeping with a system of moral beliefs about right and wrong and the resultant rightness or wrongness of certain actions. (Readers who wish to read more about ethics can find suggestions for further reading at the end of the chapter.)

Our assumptions about ethics and what constitutes ethical behaviour derive from a set of moral values and principles, by which we know the difference between right and wrong. Each of us has an internal sense of what is right and wrong, a set of constructs that we have absorbed from the culture of the society in which we live. These are not static, but change as societies change, and naturally our own attitudes and values tend to follow these changes. Ethical behaviour may be identified with the good of the individual or the group. In Western cultures the individual is prized above the larger group such as the family or clan. In other cultures ethical behaviour reflects the good of the collective rather than the individual. Variations in the values and ethics held by different cultures and societies mean that some behaviours, ideas and characteristics are seen as better or worse in different cultures. These values and moral judgements change as cultures change. Carl Rogers argued that counselling helps in the search for and identification of universal values and that people of any culture will choose options which contribute to the wellbeing of the greater social group. Human beings' need for such things as affirmation and relationships contributes to the social nature of these universal values. I am uncertain how well this optimistic view holds up today. Ethics can be very practical if used in decision making; in fact we are probably unaware of the ethical content of our everyday decision making as we have absorbed and internalised the ethical standards of our own community about the 'right way to live'. At the same time acting ethically can be full of ambiguity, complexity and never being sure you made the right choice. If ethics are used to answer the question 'What is the right thing to do?', they often fail to provide a single right answer because ethical principles often contradict rather than complement each other.

The importance of ethics to professions

Professionals of whatever discipline, need a way to demonstrate to the public that they are trustworthy; this is usually done through a profession specific code of ethics. Professional ethics exist to provide support and guidance to practitioners, and to protect the profession from behaviour that might damage the reputation and undermine its standing to the public. Professional Codes of Ethics and Standards do this by outlining the expected standards of behaviour and practice. It is not surprising that the professions have many ethical principles in common, for example, integrity, respect, competence and responsibility.

A profession is trusted to keep its members behaving ethically and act against those who breach the ethical code: that is, professions are trusted to be self-regulating. The Hippocratic Oath is one of the earliest professional ethical codes. Doctors undertake to practise medicine honestly and ethically. This means that the professional, in this case a doctor, can be trusted to act in the best interests of the client or patient.

Professional ethical codes have another function. During training they are used to socialise students into the values and culture of the particular profession, in order to strengthen the sense of identity of the profession and engender a common set of ethical values. Some professional ethical codes attempt to cover all the areas in which the profession works; others provide a framework of principles to act as guidance. Professionals are often required to make discretionary judgements and are free to do so. Ethics inform but cannot replace individual professional ethical judgement. Ethics are there to be used in the making of ethical decisions and the reflection upon and accountability for such decisions. In these circumstances the professional uses their internal ethical sense of responsibility and the ethical principles of the professional association. In such circumstances ethics provide help in reaching informed judgements that have moral authority and accountability.

Types of professional ethics

Underlying many professions' codes of ethics is a philosophical approach which creates general moral principles to identify what comprises a 'good' life. The foundation of BACP's Ethical Framework (2010) is the six moral principles of being trustworthy, autonomy, beneficence, non-maleficence, justice and self-respect. The British Psychological Society describes its ethical principles as leading to a set of values on behaviour, competence, responsibility and integrity, whereas the BACP Ethical Framework presents values as leading to the articulation of ethical principles. Although many of the professional associations' codes will have overarching similar moral principles, the translation of those into practice may vary.

There are clear differences in the language used in the ethical codes of the statutory professional regulators and those of professional associations. The codes of statutory bodies such as the Health and Care Professions Council (HCPC) uses 'must' and focuses on the duties of registrants. HCPC divides the codes into conduct, performance and ethics and describes the three as the ethical framework within which registrants must work. BACP on the other hand places performance and conduct within the overarching Ethical Framework. The codes of the voluntary professional associations such as the BACP, BPS for the most part are more aspirational and use the word 'should' rather than 'must'. There are, however, exceptions to this in the BACP *Ethical Framework for Good Practice in Counselling and Psychotherapy*, for example paragraph 17: 'Practitioners must not abuse their cleint's trust in order to gain sexual, emotional financial or any other kind of personal advantage' (BACP 2010: 7). There is currently a movement towards the incorporation of the principles and values with a set of core duties or absolutes.

Activity

Find the other examples of the use of 'must' in BACP *Ethical Framework for Good Practice in Counselling and Psychotherapy*. What do they have in common?

The importance of ethics to counselling

Ethics is regarded by many as the cornerstone of counselling, and as central to counsellors who work daily with ambiguity, uncertainty and the unknown. Ethics acts as a safety net in such uncertainty by providing an agreed framework to inform professional practice. Ethical guidelines are based in moral reasoning and require a counsellor to act with the highest ethical standards towards clients. Standing back it can be seen that ethics and counselling share some similar values and moral principles: the alleviation of distress, the enhancement of relationships, the promotion of human wellbeing, the respect for client autonomy, trustworthiness, and the commitment to maintain confidentiality.

Bond (2010) outlines six sources of counselling ethics: individual personal ethics, those of the particular theoretical model, the ethical codes of the professional association, the law of the country, moral philosophy and for some counsellors, the ethical code of the employer. From this list alone, it is possible to see the potential complexity involved in working ethically.

Activity

Ethical dilemmas

Using Bond's types of ethics that are listed in Table 6.1, try to think of examples of each where there might be conflicting ethical elements.

Example 1. You see a child in a farm shop deliberately dropping tomatoes on the ground with such force they burst. The parents are close by. What would you do?

Example 2. A client tells you something that leads you to think the child of the client's neighbour may be at risk of abuse. What would you consider and what would you do?

Table 6.1   *Possible conflicts between ethical principles*

Type of ethics	Nature of possible conflict of ethical principles
Individual personal ethics	
Ethics of theoretical model	
Ethical code of professional association	
The law of the country	
Moral philosophy	
The ethical code of an employer	

(*Source:* Bond 2010)

The phrase 'ethical mindfulness' coined by Tim Bond (2010; 2012) captures the embodiment of ethics in counselling practice. Such ethical
mindfulness in reflexive practice enables the counsellor to function in
difficult situations with conflicting and missing information and find a
way through that is in the best interests to the client. The ethics and
values of counselling are expressed by and through the counsellor, there
are no pieces of equipment or instruction manuals to use in the counselling room, even manualised therapeutic treatments are 'embodied' in the
counsellor. Counsellors need to be independent, autonomous, self-
reflective practitioners. Sometimes, the self-reflective process can take
place outside of sessions, but at other times it must happen swiftly
within a session and the reactions and reflections become part of the
session (see Chapter 7 for more on reflective practice). Counsellors have
to apply general ethical principles to particular situations. This is
demanding and challenging as it is often very difficult to reach an abso-
lute ethical position.

Counsellors use themselves in the work, without access to instruments
or devices (Woskett 1999; Rowan and Jacobs 2002). Therefore the ethics
and values are embodied in and expressed through the counsellor. This
means that a counsellor must have the capacity for self-reflection in the
moment and be able to act on those reflections, within their particular
theoretical approach (Palmer-Barnes and Murdin 2001; Stedmon and
Dallos 2009). The counsellor has to be able to make sense of what is happening in the session and to find a way to communicate that to the client

rather than being caught in whatever the dynamic of the relationship may be. In doing this, the counsellor has to pay rigorous and constant attention to boundary issues and be very aware of the risks inherent in the intimacy of the counselling relationship. At the same time as trying to work ethically and hold to the values of counselling, a counsellor must avoid the temptation to judge a client who fails to uphold similar values. This can present a very real tension in the work.

Counsellors need to develop and use an awareness of the ethical aspects of their work, beginning with the first session, when the counsellor should ask themselves 'Am I the right person to work with this client, with these issues?' An important ethical imperative is to work within your competence. (Chapter 5 looks at the 'messiah' complex.)

These paragraphs have focused on the use of ethics in the internal processes of the counsellor. The public and the client must also be considered. Clients are consumers and expect the counsellor to be competent. Professional ethical codes can help to inform the client about what constitutes good practice and when he/she is in receipt of practice that seems to be outside the ethical guidelines.

Cultural issues, exploitation and abuse of power

From within a group, it can be difficult to see and understand an outsider's view of it. Counsellors believe that counselling is a 'good thing', but this view is not shared by everyone. Counselling has been accused of undermining organised religion, removing any sense of responsibility for one's own actions and creating a society of self-centred narcissists (Dineen 1999; Smail 2001; Furedi 2004). This divergence of views over the impact of counselling on society raises the issue of the influence the counsellor can have over the client (Proctor, Cooper et al. 2000; Feltham 2010). Counselling is seen by some as the active embodiment of a set of moral values that are outside the 'mainstream capitalist society' (McLeod 2009). If counsellors socialise their clients into this value set, then counselling acts as a subversive element in capitalist society. Counselling's focus on the importance of client autonomy has led to debates on its consequences. There is an argument that therapy's emphasis on the primacy of individual needs creates a selfish society, not the more altruistic one Rogers saw. It is argued that in a secular society, each of us can decide what is morally right and good for us and the basic aim of counselling is for the client to find what is right and good for them and act upon that. Thus counselling's focus on the primacy of the individual may be unethical in terms of what society sees as morally good and right. It appears that counsellors have power for both good and bad and the client trusts us to be good. In practice the issue of the self-determination of the client or client autonomy produces ethical dilemmas, for example, whether or not to intervene with a suicidal client.

There are many ways in which a counsellor can and does influence a client, and some are difficult to avoid. It is not accidental that satisfied clients often go on to train as counsellors.

Ethics provide a useful guide to thinking about how to address the power imbalance between the professional counsellor and the client and potential abuse of the client's vulnerability. One example of this would be a counsellor who believed that he/she knew what was best for the client and tried to persuade the client of this. One of the hardest things to do is to support a client on a path you believe will lead to disappointment, failure or hurt.

It is perhaps more straightforward to think about how to avoid the exploitation of clients in terms of sexual, financial or emotional exploitation. Bond (2010) adds ideological exploitation, that is, the imposition of the counsellor's interpretation of the client's experience to validate the counsellor's belief system. McLeod (2009) also recognises a form of this process but sees it as benign, describing it as socialisation to the values of counselling, which in his view can only be beneficial.

Types of ethics

Counselling has been described as a form of applied virtue ethics which helps the client find a way to live a 'good' life (MacIntyre 2008). This raises the question of who defines what constitutes a 'good' life. It also raises the issue of how can counselling be value free – a claim that is made for it. In reality the counsellor tries very hard not to judge clients or impose upon them anything from her own moral values. This is a counsel of perfection and clients will make their own value judgements of the counsellor's value system based on appearance, dress, accent, fee etc. The 'blank screen' that analysts seek to be for their patients is in sharp contradiction to Freud's consulting room in Vienna, which is overflowing with ornaments, paintings and all sorts of items which tell the visitor a great deal about the occupant.

It has been argued that trying to be value free and non-judgemental means that the counsellor is abdicating any ethical responsibility for the counselling process and could be encouraging the client into amorality by supporting the validity of the client's internal impulses and feelings rather than the moral values of the society. Rogers denied this, relying on his belief in the social and altruistic nature of individuals. It remains an uncomfortable question for counsellors – are we unconsciously encouraging clients to conform to our social norms? In being accepting do counsellors collude in clients' views, behaviours and desires that may cause harm to another person? If a counsellor sees a client for an hour a week, what harm can a self-absorbed individual do to others in the remaining 167 hours? What is the counsellor's responsibility?

BACP ETHICAL FRAMEWORK

The BACP *Ethical Framework for Good Practice in Counselling and Psychotherapy* is a document to which most counsellors and people taking counselling skills courses will have been introduced during training. BACP has had a code of ethics since 1984 and a professional conduct process since 1986. Until 2001 this looked very different to the current Ethical Framework. There were a series of codes for counsellors, supervisors, trainers and counselling skills users. Each had a long list of behaviours which were breaches of the codes, which made it very difficult to check if you were behaving ethically against all of the codes that applied to you. It was possible to have a complaint raised against you under all four codes at once. In the later 1990s a decision was made to radically rethink the philosophical basis of ethics for counselling. This led to the current Ethical Framework which has achieved international recognition and been widely copied.

The foundation of the Ethical Framework is a moral philosophy which identifies the values and principles that should inform counselling and psychotherapy. The key principles come from well-established philosophical traditions (Engels, Engebreston et al. 2009). The values are expressed as the personal behaviours and attributes to which a counsellor should aspire to be capable of ethical good practice.

The BACP *Ethical Framework for Good Practice in Counselling and Psychotherapy* moves through values to principles to personal moral qualities. These are listed below and can also be found at www.bacp.co.uk/ ethical_framework/. These specify the personal behaviours and attributes to which a counsellor should aspire to deliver good ethical practice. The Ethical Framework includes examples of good practice to assist and support counsellors.

Values of counselling and psychotherapy

- Respecting human rights and dignity.
- Protecting the safety of clients.
- Ensuring the integrity of practitioner–client relationships.
- Enhancing the quality of professional knowledge and its application.
- Alleviating personal distress and suffering.
- Fostering a sense of self that is meaningful to the person(s) concerned.
- Increasing personal effectiveness.
- Enhancing the quality of relationships between people.
- Appreciating the variety of human experience and culture.
- Striving for the fair and adequate provision of counselling and psycho-therapy services.

Ethical principles of counselling and psychotherapy

- Being trustworthy: honouring the trust placed in the practitioner.
- Autonomy: respect for the client's right to be self-governing.
- Beneficence: a commitment to promoting the client's well-being.
- Non-maleficence: a commitment to avoiding harm to the client.
- Justice: the fair and impartial treatment of all clients and the provision of adequate services.
- Self-respect: fostering the practitioners' knowledge and care for self.

Personal moral qualities

- Empathy: the ability to communicate understating of another person's experience from that person's perspective.
- Sincerity: a personal commitment to consistency between what is professed and what is done.
- Integrity: commitment to being moral in dealing with others, personal straightforwardness, honesty and coherence.
- Resilience: the capacity to work with the client's concerns without being personally diminished.
- Respect: showing appropriate esteem to others and their understanding of themselves.
- Humility: the ability to assess accurately and acknowledge one's own strengths and weaknesses.
- Competence: the effective deployment of the skills and knowledge needed to do what is required.
- Fairness: the consistent application of appropriate criteria to inform decisions and action.
- Wisdom: possession of sound judgement that informs practice.
- Courage: the capacity to act in spite of known fears risks and uncertainty.

The counsellor is expected to use the Framework in everyday practice when reflecting upon work. It is not intended to be a 'rescue remedy' taken when faced with a dilemma or when required to make a difficult ethical decision. The Ethical Framework should not sit on a bookshelf gathering dust. It should become dog-eared from daily use.

TYPES OF ETHICAL ISSUES

General issues

This section looks briefly at some of the most common areas where ethical issues arise. One of the difficulties in getting to grips with ethics in counselling is coming to the acceptance that sometimes there is no correct ethical course of action. In these circumstances, a counsellor makes the most ethical decision possible having considered all the options, the potential outcomes and the people affected. Sometimes, the principles in the Ethical Framework appear to be in conflict with each other, for example in the case of a suicidal client, the principle of autonomy would indicate that the counsellor would not intervene to prevent the suicide. However, the principle of non-maleficence would indicate intervention to potentially preserve the client's life. At the heart of this, is the need for the counsellor to take personal responsibility for whatever ethical decision they make. Professional ethical codes and frameworks can only guide, the decision is the counsellor's own.

Influencing

Issues of this nature also raise the question of how a counsellor can be morally neutral, when dress, speech and counselling room all give messages about the counsellor. It may be difficult for the client to assert their values when it is clear that these are different to those of the counsellor. The personal beliefs of both the counsellor and client can raise ethical issues. It is straightforward to assert that the counsellor should not try to impose any personally held spiritual and religious beliefs on the client, but what if the counsellor believes that the disclosure of personal religious belief would strengthen the therapeutic alliance? Can counsellors be sure that they are not counselling clients towards the kind of social conformity that the values of counselling represent – living a 'good' life?

Activity

Look at/think about the room(s) you use for counselling, or the rooms used by a counsellor or psychotherapist you know.

- What is informative in the room about the counsellor?
- What can you learn about the counsellor from looking at that room?
- What assumptions might you make about the counsellor if you were the client? What influence might this have on the counselling?
- What could be done to minimise this?
- What might be lost in the process of doing this?

Confidentiality

Confidentiality is the first ethical issue that comes to mind when the subject of ethics is raised. Counsellors cannot promise total confidentiality to clients, and must make the limits to confidentiality clear. Some of these limits are taken for granted as part of professional practice, for example supervision, team case discussions. These may be part of practice to us, but this is not necessarily the same for clients. Clients may feel very uncomfortable at the idea of being talked about as a 'case', even if an anonymous case. How would you feel?

Client case notes may be the property of the agency, not the individual counsellor and as such a client may feel they are not therefore confidential. There are legal exemptions to confidentiality of certain things, such as terrorism, money laundering, road traffic accidents and child abuse. Again, such things may not always present in a straightforward way. If something of this nature arises, ideally the client will give consent to disclosure. If this consent is not given, the counsellor has to weigh client confidentiality against public interest. If he/she decides that disclosure is necessary, the client should be informed of it.

Informed consent

Informed consent is a term best known from medicine, where patients are given information about the potential outcomes of treatment or surgery and asked to give consent to the treatment. It is best practice in the first session to give a client full information about what counselling involves and your policies on for example, non-attendance, breaks, social meetings etc. In reality, a client may want to let go of whatever is troubling them by 'telling the story' in the first session and leave no opportunity for the giving of information. In fact to do so could damage the development of the therapeutic work. Additionally, informed consent is a more difficult issue as neither counsellor nor client know at the beginning of the work where it will lead. McLeod (2009) suggests that one simple way to address this is by having regular reviews of the work and contract and making changes if needed. Then both client and counsellor are clear.

Client assessment

Confidentiality and informed consent at times combine to present ethical issues around client assessment and, for example, informed consent when working with children and the limits of confidentiality when dealing with potential child abuse or a client seriously considering suicide. Some theoretical approaches are opposed to any kinds of formal assessment. However, all counsellors do make 'assessments' of clients and their issues in order to develop understanding, a feel for the issues and suitable responses. Feltham is clear that 'if serious suicidal impulses are in evidence then the counsellor should act swiftly to alert related professionals' (2013: 98). No one can stop another person killing themselves, and some counsellors would take a view that they should not intervene to prevent a client's suicide. I did intervene once with a suicidal client, by alerting the GP, and the client did commit suicide a few months later. I don't know if anything would have made a difference.

Issues around informed consent arise in areas such as child protection and the revelations of criminal activities, and how to balance this with the counsellor's legal obligations. Bond and Sandhu (2005) believe that all counsellors should have some understanding of the law about contracts, confidentiality, negligence, record keeping and acting as a witness in court. These topics are covered in detail in a series of books called *Legal Resources for Counsellors and Psychotherapists* that cover essential law, record keeping and confidentiality, legal issues in particular settings and therapists in court. Full details are given in the further reading at the end of the chapter.

Dual relationships

There are many possible kinds of dual relationship, but most of us immediately think of intimate personal relationships between counsellor and client. It is not unusual for a counsellor to feel sexual attraction towards a client, which in itself is not unethical. What may be unethical is the action the counsellor takes in response to those feelings (CHRE 2008). Sexual contact with a client is seen as taboo in counselling; however, there is no agreement as to whether this taboo continues after the end of the counselling relationship. Many people believe that the taboo should be life-long as they believe that the imbalance of power in the counsellor–client relationship will influence the relationship. Dual relationships can take many forms, all of which have ethical dimensions:

> Practitioners should think carefully about and exercise considerable caution before, entering into personal or business relationships with former clients and should expect to be professionally accountable if the relationship becomes detrimental to the client or the standing of the profession. (BACP 2010: 7, para. 17)

Dual relationships occur in many everyday settings, for example, in small rural communities; in schools where a counsellor is also a teacher; a university counsellor may sit on a committee with a member of staff who is a client. In circumstances where this is a likelihood, it is good practice and common sense to work out at the start of counselling how both parties want to deal with the event when and if it happens.

The use of touch in counselling

Touch is a human expression of caring in all societies, but in the counselling relationship touch is not so simple. Many counsellors are aware that touch can be an abuse of power and source of sexual gratification for the counsellor or the client. In some theoretical approaches touch is always unethical and wrong. Guidance on the subject tends to refer to clinical judgement about the appropriateness of touch, but that is not much help to the counsellor feeling the aching need of a client to be held. There is no easy answer. One useful question to ask is 'What would be the purpose and meaning of touch, to the client and to the counsellor?' McLeod provides a very useful list in his *Introduction to Counselling* (2009). In the end it depends on the clinical judgement and integrity of the counsellor.

Limits of competence

It is very easy to write that every counsellor must work within the limits of his/her competence. Sometimes it is much more difficult to put this into practice. What does a counsellor working in an agency do when she feels that a client has suddenly moved beyond her competence? If it is possible to refer to another counsellor in the agency, how does the counsellor explain this to the client without causing anxiety? What might the client understand? The client's issues/problems are too bad, too serious for the counsellor to deal with? The client has been seeing a not very competent counsellor? The client is a hopeless case? A counsellor in private practice, with a small caseload, might be tempted to carry on working with the client and try to compensate by additional supervision and reading. A significant number of complaints about counsellors involve a failure to monitor effectiveness and competence, when a counsellor has continued working with a client on issues or in a way beyond the competence of the counsellor. Research suggests that counsellors are poor at hearing clients express dissatisfaction with therapy and many complaints involve poor practice. However, some research suggests that therapists do recognise their own failings (Braun and Roussos 2012).

Record keeping

The area of record keeping is complex and counsellors must abide by the legal requirements of for example, the Data Protection Act. Protocols on record keeping can vary with agencies, but whatever these are, clients need to give consent to record keeping and have the right to see what is written about them. In terms of access to records, counsellors have the same rights as a doctor or social worker and a search warrant signed by a circuit judge is required. A useful book on this subject is *Confidentiality and Record*

Keeping in Counselling and Psychotherapy (Bond and Mitchels 2008), one in the series of Legal Resources for counsellors and psychotherapists.

Ethics in specific contexts

It is the case that the counselling room is the main place where counsellors use ethics and are faced with ethical dilemmas. However, some distinct areas justify special mention: three are touched on in this section – research and on-line work and social media.

Research   The major ethical issues which arise in research are informed consent and the confidentiality of research data and the care of informants and the self-care of the researcher/counsellor. These are especially important in research which includes client experience (West 2002). Universities require students to submit research proposals for ethical consent, and the consent forms provide a helpful guide for issues to consider. The difficulty of obtaining and maintaining true informed consent in the counselling relationship has already been mentioned, but there are other areas to take into account in research. Confidentiality of the research data is one area where ethics needs to be carefully thought through and processes agreed with informants. Data needs to be collected and usually this is by taped interview. Such data will be transcribed, but if a transcriber is employed this could be a breach of confidentiality. Data analysis can take many forms, but it is not unusual to have a third party involved to verify the accuracy of ratings and coding. In writing up research care has to be taken that informants cannot be identified, and that they consent to what is to be written about them, if that was the original agreement.

Once written up, research findings need an audience, and this can be an international one. It is very difficult to avoid a creeping objectification of informants during this process. It is good practice to agree all of these issues in a research contract at the start, but the point of some research is that we do not know the outcomes at the start, otherwise there would be little point in the research. It is also difficult to know the impact of the research on informants and researcher. The research may also have an impact on people wider than the researcher and informants, for example the families of both, and employers; Swain (1996) lists up to 14 different groups who may be affected by research. BACP's *Ethical Guidelines for Researching Counselling and Psychotherapy* provide guidance and support to any counsellor embarking on research (Bond 2004).

The counsellor carrying out research, especially if this is in the area of client experience, has to stay in the role of researcher and be aware of the temptation to move into the counselling role (Gabriel and Casemore 2009). This can be very challenging if informants know that the researcher's primary role is that of counsellor. Learning of bad experiences and trauma and not responding as a counsellor can cause stress and self-doubt in the researcher. Being an informant can also re-open old hurt and distress. The counsellor/researcher has an ethical obligation to keep this possibility in mind and ask him/herself what would be the likely impact of this methodology on the informant. Is that ethically justifiable? Am I exploiting my informants?

On-line counselling   On-line counselling raises some specific ethical issues on safety and confidentiality. It is very difficult to know for certain the identity of an on-line client and therefore it is difficult to know if the client is a minor.

A counsellor working on-line, needs to be aware of the potential problems of professional jurisdiction. It can be difficult to know which country the client is resident in. This is important as in the case of a complaint, the rules and regulation will be those of the country of the client not the counsellor. For example, what in the United Kingdom would be ordinary counselling, for example working with a client with diagnosed depression, in some European countries is restricted to state registered psychologists and psychotherapists. Mandatory reporting of such things as terrorism also varies in different countries. This area is covered in far more detail in the books suggested for further reading at the end of this chapter.

Social media   Many of us use social media in our private/personal lives, but are careful about self-disclosure in the counselling room. In this we may be naive, for little is really private if someone wants to find out about you, including clients. For example, anyone can find videos of me on road racing websites and YouTube. This might lead a client to doubt my ability to be accepting of their less active life style. This can also leave a counsellor open to 'trolls' and unhappy clients. Social media exposes the gossamer thin divide between the personal and professional world and as a result can lead to a counsellor facing charges of bringing the profession into disrepute. People have turned to Human Rights legislation over this ethical blurring between professional reputation and the right to a personal life.

SUPERVISION

Supervision is covered in Chapter 8 on the counselling profession and careers in counselling. This section considers the role of ethics in supervision. The term is often misunderstood and taken to mean that counsellors must be overseen in their work and cannot work independently. Despite a search for an alternative phrase, such as 'consultative support', or the change of title from supervisor to professional mentor (Bond and Mitchels 2008: 43) the term supervision has stuck and counsellors have to try to explain what it means.

Supervision supports ethical practice and protects ethical standards on both an individual and profession-wide level. It provides professional support for the counsellor but it also has a protective function for the client. Throughout the professional life of a counsellor supervision is the main quality assurance mechanism of the profession.

Supervision, by its very existence widens the confidentiality of client information and therefore must be included in the informed consent a client gives at the start of counselling. This is an area where it is advisable to think through issues in detail: Will the client's name be used? Can the client refuse to be discussed in supervision? Will you tell the client what was discussed about them in supervision? Can the client complain about the supervisor? Any written communications come under Data Protection Legislation and clients need to give explicit consent and have the right to see what was written about them. Both counsellor and supervisor need to keep this in mind. It may become apparent that the supervisor knows one of the clients being presented. What is the ethical course of action?

The supervisor is required to weigh and balance ethical issues in the responsibility he/she holds for the supervisee, the clients, in some cases the employing agency and the standards and reputation of counselling in general. At the same time she must respect the autonomy of the supervisee and her own integrity. It has been observed that ethical issues tend to arise during supervision, rather than be brought openly and directly by the supervisee. This places a responsibility on the supervisor to be alert at all times to the possible ethical dimensions of each session, and exposes the supervisor to accountability for the work of his/her supervisees. The recommendations of the Francis report on Stafford Hospital may lead to an increase in this type of responsibility (Francis 2013).

Another ethical issue which arises in supervision is the boundary between supervision and counselling. The focus of supervision is the work with the client, not the personal needs of the counsellor, but at times the work brings the counsellor's own needs to the forefront. When this happens it is the ethical responsibility of the supervisor to ensure that the counsellor recognises and accepts the need for self-care. Supervisors need clear explicit contracts about this and supervisees must understand the need for clear boundaries or they may feel abandoned.

When things go wrong

Given the large number of counselling sessions that take place each week, it is reasonable to assume that quite a few things go wrong quite often – most of which are never heard about. Dissatisfied clients just don't turn up again. Outcome research has found that a percentage of clients become worse after therapy, with percentages ranging from 5 to 10 per cent, but this has not been correlated to practice that would give rise to complaints. Relatively few formal complaints are made about counsellors and there is little research to fill in the gaps. This section presents an overview of what goes wrong and what can be learnt, using research findings (Garrett and Davis 1998; Symons 2012) and information on complaints from one professional association – BACP (Khele, Symons et al. 2008; Symons, Khele et al. 2010).

This is a difficult area to consider and research suggests that counsellors have a Polyanna-ish view and tend to attribute poor therapy to factors to do with the client rather than their own practice (Symons 2012). Things go wrong from the perspective of the client, counsellor, supervisor, student or manager. A client may be unhappy with or dissatisfied with the counselling he/she has received. A counsellor may be unhappy with the processes and management of the service in which they work. A supervisor may consider that the counsellor is working beyond her competence with a particular client and refusing to make an onward referral. A student may feel intimidated into a sexual relationship with a trainer. A manager of a service may have concerns about the quality of a counsellor's work or relationship with clients. Each of these concerns has ethical dimensions and each topic has been the subject of complaints.

Professional associations such as BACP will expect that all routes available have been followed before the issue is taken up by the professional association. For example, that the student has used the college or university's complaint processes; that the manager has addressed the issue with the counsellor and the supervisor. These are often administrative processes and are not written in terms of overt breaches of ethical standards, although such breaches may form part of the complaint. Sometimes, there is inconsistency. For example, it is a breach of BACP's Ethical Framework for a tutor to have a sexual relationship with a student on his/her counselling training course and would come under the Heads of Complaint in the BACP Professional Conduct Procedure. In higher education institutions, while not encouraged, such relationships will not lead to disciplinary actions if the tutor concerned ensures that he/she has no part in assessing the student's work.

Counselling is not subject to statutory regulation, which means there is no legal way to stop someone working as a counsellor and using the title counsellor. (The same is true of psychotherapy and psychoanalysis.) As a result, the impact of an upheld complaint against a counsellor depends upon the reputation and standing of the professional association with the public and employers.

There are two ways in which BACP receives complaints, through the Professional Conduct Procedure (PCP) and under Article 12.6 of the Memoranda and Articles of the Association. Anyone can make a complaint against a member of BACP in the Professional Conduct Procedure under the headings of professional misconduct, professional malpractice and bringing the profession into disrepute (full details of the PCP can be found in www.bacp.co.uk/ethical_framework/). If an allegation is very serious it can be heard under Article 12.6 of the Memoranda and Articles of the Association and requires a higher burden of proof than in the Professional Conduct Procedure. The only outcome of an upheld 12.6 complaint is expulsion from membership. In some cases, the matter is so serious that BACP itself brings a case against a member.

What are the subjects of complaints?   In two surveys of BACP complaints from 1996 to 2007 the most common grounds for complaint were boundary issues (39 per cent) including confidentiality, dual relationships and endings; misuse of power by the therapist (25 per cent) that harmed the client; sexual misconduct with both current and ex-clients (14 per cent); negligence and dishonesty (10 per cent each) (Khele, Symons et al. 2008; Symons, Khele et al. 2010).

Many of these examples of unethical behaviour can arise from the counsellor not thinking things through carefully with the Ethical Framework in mind. The counsellor may believe that the hand on the knee shows empathy and the client may experience it as an intimate intrusion and throw into doubt his/her belief in the counsellor's trustworthiness. The notices pages of the BACP Professional Conduct website contain the findings of cases and provide many examples from which we can all learn.

Who complains?   A significant number of complaints made to BACP are made by members against other members, students against trainers, supervisors against supervisees and the other way round, and therapist against therapist. Almost half of complaints against counsellors over the delivery of therapy were from lay clients, that is, people outside of the profession. Although increasing, the number of complaints from clients is small, when considered against the number of counselling sessions that happen every week.

Who doesn't complain?   Counsellors, trainers, supervisors and trainees have an ethical responsibility to be aware of harmful or abusive practice whether as recipient or observer. It is easy to state that this is an ethical responsibility for the individual to take action and report the behaviour, and some people do. But it appears that more do not. One reason for taking no action is that trainees and supervisees at the start of a career fear that making a complaint would have a negative impact on their future career. It has been suggested that a natural position for a counsellor to take is to try to understand the behaviour before taking action.

Research into why clients did not complain identified multiple factors that combined to keep clients silent (Symons 2012). Many of the complaints would have been about poor practice rather than manipulative abuse and clients felt the formal procedures were too weighty. Such clients would rather the counsellor said sorry in a non-confrontational setting. Others lacked information and the confidence to make a complaint. Some retained a sense of loyalty to the therapist and took some responsibility on themselves for what went wrong rather than see that responsibility as resting with the counsellor. It seems clear that professional associations could do much more to enable and empower clients to complain. Clients seem to give counsellors the benefit of the doubt when they are unhappy about something in therapy and counsellors accept it at face value.

While researching for this book and developing the BACP Certificate of Proficiency a characteristic of counsellors has begun to emerge, that counsellors accept client deference, and seem unable to hear negative comments from clients. This is supported in the research (Symons 2012). As Lambert (2013) shows, counsellors prefer to have a positive view of themselves, consistently rating themselves as better than colleagues. In the BACP Certificate of Proficiency candidates do not choose options that show doubt or a negative aspect of the counsellor but do choose options with positive feedback from clients regardless of the circumstances.

Who is complained against?   There has been some research in this area, but it is difficult to draw any firm conclusions. It has been suggested that person-centred counsellors are more likely to be subject to complaints about boundaries and the psychodynamic counsellors are more likely to receive complaints about behaviour perceived as intimidating. Other studies suggest a tendency to narcissism and impulsive behaviour may make a therapist more vulnerable to complaints. A more reliable finding is that across the helping professions, men in mid to late career are the group more likely to be the subject of formal complaint (Garrett and Davis 1998).

Sanctions   In the BACP process, if a complaint is upheld normally sanctions will be imposed with a timeframe for meeting them. The purpose is not punishment or to provide specific redress but to enhance the protection of the public who enter counselling, to promote confidence in the profession and to provide learning. At the individual level, the aim is to assist the member to understand what went wrong and to take steps to learn from this to ensure nothing similar happens again. Sanctions therefore are usually educative and developmental and may involve training, supervision and written reflection on the learning. One example of a sanction would be that the counsellor was required to submit evidence of learning from and understanding of the issues raised in the case. Another might require the counsellor to change their understanding of dual relationship and where responsibility rests between counsellor and client. It is not unusual for a member to be interviewed by the Sanctions panel after a set period of time or required to submit evidence of learning and changed practice. There are of course sanctions that remove membership. This is a difficult area for counselling organisations. As already stated, no one can be prevented from advertising and working as a counsellor. The purpose of Professional Conduct Procedures is to protect the public. Is that best done be expulsion from membership, when the individual can go on working and clients have no redress? Or should the professional association attempt to support the counsellor to improve their practice? There is no good answer that fits all, and members who do not comply with the sanctions have their membership withdrawn.

How to avoid things going wrong

By this stage any person-centred or psychodynamic middle-aged male reader who looked at himself in the mirror this morning may be wondering how long he has before he receives a complaint!

All counsellors have the capacity to work ethically and deliver good enough practice to clients, and almost all counsellors do this. The rate of complaint against BACP members is 1:1,000–1,500, which is low in comparison to other professions. The complex reasons why clients do not complain means that there is no room for complacency. DNA (did not attend) figures almost certainly include a number of clients who feel let down, disappointed, failures or exploited.

Counselling calls for constant reflection, using the Ethical Framework self-reflection and discussion with colleagues and supervisors. The self-reflective counsellor will recognise that he/she will not be the right counsellor for every client. With some clients it will be a struggle to be good enough and not always a success. This may lead to a referral to a colleague. There will be others with whom the alliance will 'fly'. Reflection will also raise awareness of ruptures in the therapeutic alliance and enable the counsellor to address these (Coutinho, Ribeiro et al. 2011). What matters is that the same level of self-reflection happens with all these clients.

Counsellors know what counselling is, clients often do not and as a result do not know if their unease or discomfort is part of the process or the result of poor or abusive practice. Many complaints could be avoided if clear contracts are established at the start of counselling and that counsellor and client also regularly review the work and re-negotiate the contract if necessary. This might also help to reduce client deference. I remember the shock I felt when a client said in a review 'I know you are trying to help me, but I don't like you. You're thin.' I would like to write that I used this to help both of us gain insight and have a good outcome, but I didn't. I wasn't good enough to work well with her.

Counsellors seem to be vulnerable to poor practice and therefore complaints when there is stress in personal life and a mixing up of the personal and professional. The endless relationship building and ending of counselling drains energy and emotion. There needs to be re-charging in private life that cannot happen if the two are intertwined. This is when and how boundaries are broken. This makes self-care an ethical imperative (BACP 2010: 8, para. 40, 10, paras 64–5; Skovholt and Trotter-Mathison 2011). If you don't care for yourself, how can you care for another person?

CONCLUSION

It seems that the things that can go wrong are usually the result of the behaviour of the counsellor. There are some counsellors who intentionally set out to get their own needs met by clients. These counsellors are not going to read, reflect on and use any ethical framework. A second group of counsellors (probably the majority who find themselves the subject of complaints) unintentionally harm clients through poor practice and unethical behaviour, perhaps as a result of poor training, poor or little supervision and a lack of reflective practice. It seems that this poor harmful practice is under reported in terms of formal complaints. Some counsellors seem to find it difficult to hear negative comments and this combined with client deference can lead to the continuation of poor practice. In such circumstances, when a client has expressed some negative comment the BACP Ethical Framework suggests that 'An apology may be the appropriate response' (2010: 8, para. 42).

There is a move in all professions towards encouraging professionals to monitor and evaluate practice throughout a whole career. Counselling is at the forefront of that move with its emphasis on self-reflection, supervision and the Ethical Framework.

FURTHER READING ON ETHICS

Blackburn, S. (2001). *A Very Short Introduction to Ethics*. Oxford, Oxford University Press.
Blackburn, S. (2002). *Being Good: A Short Introduction to Ethics*. Oxford, Oxford University Press.

Driver, J. (2007). *Ethics: the Fundamentals*. Oxford, Blackwell Publishing.
MacIntyre, A. (1966). *A Short History of Ethics. A History of Moral Philosophy from the Homeric Age to the 20th Century*. London, Routledge.
MacIntyre, A. (2008). 'Virtues, values and the good life. Virtue Ethics and its implications for counselling.' *Counselling and Values* **52**(2): 150–71.
Panza, C. and A. Potthast (2010). *Ethics for Dummies*. Hoboken, Wiley Publishing.

FURTHER READING ON COUNSELLING AND THE LAW

Bond, T. and A. Sandhu (2005). *Therapists in Court: Providing Evidence and Supporting Witnesses*. London, BACP/Sage.
Bond, T. and B. Mitchels (2008). *Confidentiality and Record Keeping in Counselling and Psychotherapy*. London, BACP/Sage.
Jenkins, P. (2007). *Counselling, Psychotherapy and the Law*. Second Edition. London, Sage.
Mitchels, B. and T. Bond (2010). *Essential Law for Counsellors and Psychotherapists*. London, BACP/Sage.
Mitchels, B. and T. Bond (2011). *Legal Issues Across Counselling and Psychotherapy Settings*. London, BACP/Sage.

FURTHER READING ON ONLINE COUNSELLING

Anthony, K. and S. Goss (2009). *Guidelines for Online Counselling and Psychotherapy*. Third Edition, including *Guidelines for Online Supervision*. Rugby, BACP.
Anthony, K. and D.M. Nagel (2010). *Therapy Online: A Practical Guide*. London, Sage.
Jones, G. and A. Stokes (2009). *On-line Counselling: A Handbook for Practitioners*. Basingstoke, Palgrave Macmillan.

REFERENCES

BACP (2010). *Ethical Framework for Good Practice in Counselling and Psychotherapy* (T. Bond). Lutterworth, BACP.
Bond, T. (2004). *Ethical Guidelines for Researching Counselling and Psychotherapy*. Lutterworth, BACP.
Bond, T. (2010). *Standards and Ethics for Counselling in Action*. London, Sage.

Bond, T. (2012). 'Ethical imperialism or ethical mindfulness? Rethinking ethical review for social sciences.' *Research Ethics* **8**(2): 97–112.

Bond, T. and A. Sandhu (2005). *Therapists in Court: Providing Evidence and Supporting Witnesses*. London, BACP/Sage.

Braun, M. and A. J. Roussos (2012). 'Psychotherapy Researchers: reported misbehaviours and opinions.' *Journal of Empirical Research on Human Research Ethics* **7**(5): 25–9.

CHRE (2008). *Clear Sexual Boundaries Between Healthcare Professionals and Patients: Responsibilities of Healthcare Professionals*. London, CHRE (Council for Healthcare Regulatory Excellence).

Coutinho, J., E. Ribeiro, C. Hill and J. Safran (2011). 'Therapists' and clients' experiences of alliance rupture: A qualitative study.' *Psychotherapy Research* **21**(5): 525–40.

Davies, M. (2007). *Boundaries in Counselling and Psychotherapy*. Twickenham, Athena Press.

Dineen, T. (1999). *Manufacturing Victims: What the Psychology Industry is Doing to People*. London, Constable.

Engels, D. W., K. Engebreston, et al. (2009). 'Kitchener's Principle Ethics: implications for counselling practice and research.' *Counselling and Values* **53**(1): 67–78.

Feltham, C. (2010). *Critical Thinking in Counselling and Psychotherapy*. London, Sage.

Feltham, C. (2013). *Counselling and Counselling Psychology: A Critical Examination*. Ross-on-Wye, PCCS Books.

Francis, R. (2013). *Independent Inquiry into Care Provided by Mid Staffordshire NHS Foundation Trust January 2005–March 2009*. London, House of Commons.

Furedi, F. (2004). *Therapy Culture*. London, Routledge.

Gabriel, L. and R. Casemore (Eds) (2009). *Relational Ethics in Practice: Narratives from Counselling and Psychotherapy*. Hove, Routledge.

Garrett, T. and J. D. Davis (1998). 'The prevalence of sexual contact between British clinical psychologists and their patients.' *Clinical Psychoogy and Psychotherapy* **5**: 253–263.

Hinshelwood, R. D. (1997). *Therapy as Coercion. Does Psychoanalysis Differ from Brainwashing?* London, Karnac Books.

Khele, S., C. Symons, et al. (2008). 'An analysis of complaints to the BACP, 1996–2006.' *Counselling and Psychotherapy Research* **8**(2): 124–32.

Lambert, M. J. (2013). *Keynote Address*. BACP Research Conference, Coventry, BACP.

MacIntyre, A. (2008). 'Virtues, values and the good life: virtue ethics and its implications for counselling.' *Counselling and Values* **52**(2): 150–71.

Masson, J. (1990). *Against Therapy*. London, Harper-Collins.

McLeod, J. (2009). *An Introduction to Counselling*. Maidenhead, Open University Press.

Palmer-Barnes, F. and L. Murdin (Eds) (2001). *Values and Ethics in the Practice of Psychotherapy and Counselling*. Buckingham, Open University Press.

Proctor, G., M. Cooper, et al. (Eds) (2000). *Politicizing the Person-centred Approach: An Agenda for Social Change*. Ross on Wye, PCCS Books.

Rowan, J. and M. Jacobs (2002). *The Therapist's Use of Self*. Oxford, Oxford University Press.

Sands, A. (2000). *Falling for Therapy*. Basingstoke, Macmillan.

Skovholt, T. and M. Trotter-Mathison (2011). *The Resilient Practitioner. Burnout Prevention and Self-care Strategies for Counselors, Therapists and Health Professionals*. New York, London, Routledge Taylor and Francis Group.

Smail, D. (2001). *The Nature of Unhappiness*. London, Robinson.

Stedmon, J. and R. Dallos (Eds) (2009). *Reflective Practice in Psychotherapy and Counseling*. New York, Oxford University Press.

Swain, R. (1996). 'Ethical codes, confidentiality and the law.' *The Irish Journal of Psychology* **17**(2): 95–109.

Symons, C. (2012). *Complaints and Complaining in Counselling and Psychotherapy: Organisational and Client Perspectives*. Leicester, University of Leicester.

Symons, C., S. Khele, et al. (2010). 'Allegations of serious professional misconduct: An analysis of the BACP 4.6 cases, 1998–2007.' *Counselling and Psychotherapy Research* **11**(4): 257–65.

West, W. (2002). 'Some ethical dilemmas in counselling and in counselling research.' *British Journal of Guidance and Counselling* **30**(3): 261–8.

Wood, D. (1993). *The Power of Words. Uses and abuses of Talking Treatments*. London, Mind Publications.

Woskett, V. (1999). *The Therapeutic Use of Self: Counselling Practice Research and Supervision*. London, Routledge.

7 UNDERSTANDING RESEARCH IN COUNSELLING

INTRODUCTION

Some readers at this point may think 'I won't ever do any research' and be tempted to skip the whole chapter. Please don't. The interesting findings and examples in this book about ethics, counsellor resilience and failings have all come from research. The interviews I have conducted for this book, themselves represent a form of research. This is not a chapter on research methodology. It does not teach the reader how to conduct research. Books on this subject are referenced throughout the chapter and are to be found in the References section at the end of the chapter.

The chapter has three aims. The first is to consider some of the issues that research may pose for counsellors and counselling and the reasons for these, including the politics of research. The second is to describe some of the research that is useful to counsellors. Finally, it touches on reflective practice, by which counsellors and other helping professionals explore and enhance their understanding. The hope is that the chapter will provide enough information for you to be able to come to your own decisions about the place of research in counselling. My own view is that the future for counselling and counsellors is research-informed practice. Unless counsellors can provide credible evidence that counselling produces good outcomes for clients, then promoting counselling is no better than selling snake oil. The research referred to in this chapter includes research from all the psychological therapies, that is, counselling, psychotherapy and some forms of psychology.

Research takes many forms, but all research comprises organised systematic ways to explore and gain new knowledge and understanding of the subject(s) of the research. A theory may be tested to see if it holds up under systematic scrutiny, a theoretical approach may be tested to see if it produces beneficial change in clients with a particular problem or condition.

An individual or an organisation may be the subject of an in-depth case study.

The goals of research are to discover if the findings of the research are valid, reliable and generalisable.

Validity means the research and the results must be valid, that is that the research has done what it said it would do in the way that it said.

> Example: The research is looking at the home and away performance of Premier League football teams. It would not be valid to include performances in the FA Cup as some of these games will be against non-premier league teams.

Reliablity means if other people carried out the same research they would get the same results.

> Example: If you go regularly to the same restaurant and so do your friends, and the food is always good. The restaurant is reliable.

Generalisability. A further goal of much research is to produce results that can be generalised. This means that the findings from the research can be used in broader contexts and achieve equivalent outcomes.

> Example: Having read the example about the restaurant, would you expect to have a good meal in any restaurant? No – because you cannot generalise from one restaurant to all others. But, if the restaurant is one of a chain, you might reasonably expect the same standard in other branches. So you could generalise about a chain of restaurants.

There is a major division in the methodologies used between qualitative and quantitative research. Qualitative research uses language rather than numbers and explores the processes and perceptions of counsellor and client and the outcomes arising from that. Quantitative research tends to use numbers, and involve large numbers of subjects and the findings are often written as statistics and conclusions that can be applied wider than the specific research project, that is they can be generalised. Such research may use questionnaires and rating forms. Quantitative researchers may have a different philosophical base, one that believes in the existence of objective truth(s) that can be tested and proved. Counsellors tend to be drawn towards qualitative research as the values seem more congruent. For example, counsellors accept each client's view of reality, rather than trying to help the client see the one true reality. Readers wishing to explore this further should read John McLeod's *Introduction to Counselling* (2009: 584).

Activity

Which of the following would you choose to understand the incidence of unprotected sexual intercourse among under-age girls? What guided your choice?

1 A case study of four under-age pregnant teenagers.
2 An on-line questionnaire linked to a teen magazine.

RESEARCH IN THE PSYCHOLOGICAL THERAPIES

The earliest and best known kind of research in the psychological therapies is the case study, exemplified by Freud's case studies of his patients, for example Little Hans and the Wolf Man. The findings of a case study on client A cannot be applied with any confidence or credibility to clients B, C and D. Therefore, in research terms such case studies are not reliable and cannot be used to develop generalisations. However, Freud used his case studies to develop the theoretical basis of psychoanalysis.

In 1967 Gordon Paul wrote a much-quoted sentence about research into the psychological therapies: 'What treatment by whom is most effective for this client with that specific problem and under which set of circumstances?' (Paul 1967: 111, quoted in Cooper 2008: 58). In the twenty-first century these remain the questions counselling research seeks to answer. Research forms part of a triangle with theory and practice that ideally blend together in the counsellor, illustrated in Figure 7.1. There is logic to this, as each part informs and learns from the other two. In reality, while theory and practice are integrated in training and clinical work, research

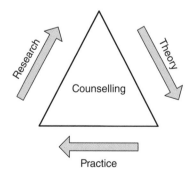

Figure 7.1 *The equilateral triangle of counselling*

often remains a weak third part, and as a result there remains a gap between research and practice.

One reason for this may be that recently research into the psychological therapies has focused on the cost effectiveness of interventions. This can elicit a hostile response in many counsellors, well expressed in Oscar Wilde's phrase about 'knowing the price of everything and the value of nothing'. Much counselling research is very practical in its objectives: it aims to find out what works and who it works for. Counsellors can use these findings to provide a better service to clients. Counselling research can also be part of everyday practice, for example session-by-session evaluation by both counsellor and client to produce practice-based evidence for studies in effectiveness.

THE ROLE OF RESEARCH IN COUNSELLING

There are disagreements and debates over the role of research in counselling and the forms that research should take. Research can appear to be an academic activity far removed from the human intimacy of the counselling interaction. But, as Cooper (2008) says, 'the facts are friendly', the research undertaken tells us that counselling works; over 40 per cent of clients improve and this improvement is sustained for up to two years. This can be overlooked in the issues raised about counselling research.

Counsellors' issues about research

There are objections to some research methodologies, such as making clients the subjects of research, especially research that calls for session-by-session evaluations carried out in the sessions. This requirement is not restricted to research studies but is an increasingly common requirement in practice, for example in IAPT (Improving Access to Psychological Therapies) services. Counsellors have concerns that this interferes with the development of the therapeutic alliance and interrupts the therapeutic work and that it objectifies the client. Clients on the other hand, appear to welcome the systematic way to see the progress made, or the barriers to progress. Counsellors working in services that require session-by-session evaluation and measurement have found ways to integrate this into the therapeutic process.

A further argument is that counsellor and client know what things worked well and what things did not. They do not need to fill in forms to tell them this. Therapists of all theoretical approaches believe that their own experience with clients and clinical judgement guides their work more than any research. However, research with clients on their experience and evaluation of therapy does not appear to support this (Watson and Rennie 1994; Timulak 2010; Bachelor 2013).

Another objection is to the way in which theoretical approaches are formatted into intervention manuals to which counsellors must adhere for the purposes of the research. This seems to be a way to control and restrict creativity and discount the uniqueness of the client. This opposition tends to be towards the traditional research model of randomised controlled trials which are described on pages 147–8.

It can be difficult to access research, both physically and intellectually. Professional associations publish research journals, for example BACP publishes *Counselling and Psychotherapy Research* (CPR) and such journals are usually free to members. To get a broad picture of up-to-date research a counsellor would have to belong to several organisations or subscribe to several journals, only to find perhaps one article a quarter that had real relevance to his/her work. It may be possible to read these journals in a local university or college library, if counselling is taught there.

The second access issue is the way in which research is written sometimes might as well be in a foreign language. Research is written for publication in the language that is conventionally accepted for peer reviewed journals. Glossaries such as the one in Cooper's book help, but the terminology can be a barrier (Cooper 2008). The challenge therefore, is to make research accessible and meaningful to counsellors while retaining its academic validity.

The positives of research

The large numbers of counsellors who are interested and involved in research outweigh these doubts and negative views of research. BACP has had a number of Practice Research Networks (PRNs) for members since 1999. Members of a PRN are a 'group of practising clinicians that cooperates to collect data and conduct research studies' in typical clinical settings. Because network members are both practitioners and researchers the PRN helps to promote the dissemination and transfer of research findings into practice (www.bacp.co.uk/research/).

Professional bodies also hold research conferences, BAC's first research conference was in 1994. It was the enthusiasm and buzz of this conference that led me into research. I wanted to be part of the excitement of 'finding out things'. In this research and counselling share a common motivation – to find out more about human beings: curiosity about how people are. How do we become as we are? What brings about change? Does theory A work with everyone or just some people? If so, who and why? At a level of everyday practice this may be discussed in supervision and case discussion groups, with questions such as, 'Why do I do better work with this sort of client?'

Reflective practice

Reflective practice is one of the fundamental elements of counselling, in training, personal development, client work and supervision. It could have been positioned in several other chapters in this book. I have chosen to put it in the Research chapter in order to show the shared principles between reflective practice and research. Both are open to uncertainty, to new knowledge and understanding. Both challenge existing views and beliefs and incorporate and adapt to new knowledge: 'Reflection-in-action links the art of practice in uncertainty and uniqueness to the scientists' art of "research"' (Schon 1983: 69). Du Plock considers that 'therapists who take reflexivity seriously are ideally positioned to generate forms of research grounded in first-person experience and naive inquiry' (Bager-Charleson 2010: 122). Indeed, one area of research, auto-ethnography, is built from reflective practice (Etherington 2004).

Reflective practice is not unique to the psychological therapies, it is a common feature of all professions (Schon 1983). Reflective practice when considered with specific reference to counselling uses many of these concepts of 'reflection-in-action' and 'reflection-on-action'. Reflective practice encourages counsellors to stand back and try to identify their cultural and personal assumptions and meanings, vulnerabilities and tacit knowledge. The aim is a greater degree of objectivity, while recognising that objectivity can never be achieved. Such reflective practice will open up new and unexpected understandings and may lead to changes in basic assumptions and values. A reflective practitioner will feel loss when such changes happen but also an acceptance and excitement of the new.

One of the key principles in reflective practice is that the professional does not have a monopoly over accurate knowledge and understanding. Thus the client also has knowledge, assumptions and culturally derived meanings of equal value (Schon 1983; Kim and Cardemi 2012). Bager-Charleson suggests that it is helpful to think of reflective practice as having three distinct foci – the counsellor's own biases and vulnerabilities, the dynamic of relationships with clients, which she names 'reflexive self-awareness', for example counter-transference, and the relationship with our culture and society (2010).

Research into clients' experience can help a counsellor think differently about some of their own clients, by better understanding the issues or different ways of addressing issues. One of the benefits is that research can include the experiences of many more clients than the case load of a single counsellor. Research can help with where to start, the likelihood of things happening and can help increase a counsellor's knowledge and under-standing of the client's experience and views. At a more practical level, having the evidence that counselling works and in a cost effective way can influence funding and jobs.

Every counsellor can use research findings to inform their own practice and some counsellors will become active researchers. Every year, groups of students present their current research at the BACP Research confer-ence, and each one has created a new piece of knowledge to the field. Talking to these students and hearing about their research, I am always struck by the journey and the enthusiasm they have, and the joy in what they have explored and discovered.

The politics of research

A counsellor works in the intimacy of one-to-one sessions, but counsel-ling, as a profession, moves in a much larger external world. Counselling and the BACP are engaged in the task of gaining public recognition and acceptance. One goal is recognition as a profession on a par with psychol-ogy for example. This calls for academic credibility and professional respect. One of the ways to achieve this is by the production of high-quality research in the forms accepted by such organisations as NICE (National Institute for Health and Care Excellence) and published in peer reviewed journals of international standing.

The most influential research in the psychological therapies at pre-sent are Randomised Controlled Trials (RCTs) to demonstrate efficacy. RCTs began as tests for medical treatments, in particular for drugs. In these trials patients were given either the drug or a harmless inert sub-stance which looked the same; a placebo. This is difficult to replicate exactly in trials of the psychological therapies, yet RCTs dominate the evidence used to produce NICE guidelines for the psychological thera-pies. This is quantitative research that leads to the evidence-based practice in the form of NICE Guidelines. This has led to bitter disputes, as the evidence to date supports one particular theoretical approach – Cognitive Behavioural Therapy. There are relatively few RCTs of other theoretical approaches (Cooper and Reeves 2012). This is partly because of philosophical opposition to the methodology and partly because of the costs of running such trials. It is estimated that one RCT costs about £1 million.

NICE for England, Wales and Northern Ireland and SIGN for Scotland analyse the research evidence and produce guidelines for medical treat-ments that are effective in terms of outcomes and cost. As the remit of NICE evolved to include mental health conditions and therefore psychological therapy, the evidence considered remained the same. This means that the effectiveness of counselling is assessed using the same methodology that is used for drugs. This favouring of a particular form of research evidence has been criticised by many in the field of psychological therapy, for example the major psychological therapy organisations have argued for NICE to change its approach to guideline development for the psychological therapies. It appears that the evidence base may be under review. In the past both BACP and UKCP have submitted evidence to Parliamentary Select Committees on the subject in an attempt to persuade NICE to widen the evidence base for guideline development to include the range of robust research methods, rather than saying one method is de facto better than another.

The drug is a fixed element in an RCT, the same for everyone who takes it. If the therapist is equated to the drug, then clearly there will be uncontrolled individual differences which will invalidate the trial. This has been addressed by trialling specific theoretical techniques and making these into manuals of treatment to which all the therapists in a trial must adhere. This is an attempt to remove the variable presented by the therapists. Many of the counselling and psychotherapy organisations have and continue to argue for revision to the hierarchy of evidence to give more weight to practice-based evidence on the grounds that such manualised treatments do not translate into everyday practice. However the current NICE hierarchy of evidence gives little weight to such evidence.

NICE uses what is called 'a hierarchy of evidence' in the evaluation process:

Grade 1: High-quality meta-analyses of RCTs and RCTs with a low risk of bias.

Grade 2: High-quality systematic reviews of case control or cohort studies.

Grade 3: Non-analytic studies of case reports.

Grade 4: Expert opinion and formal consensus.

This may look reasonable, but there are indicators that this approach can have weaknesses. Meta-analyses of research studies have shown evidence that 'researcher allegiance' impacts on the findings (Wampold 2001). For example, a psychodynamic-oriented researcher will make a favourable finding of the outcomes of a trial of psychodynamic therapy. A researcher of a different orientation will produce results less positive for a psychodynamic approach. In RCT research with clients, some people argue that the methodology does not take into account the uniqueness of each client or the dynamics of the relationships. This argument is countered if the RCT has a large number of subjects, or a meta-analysis of RCTs is carried out, then the outcomes will be valid and reliable.

In addition, there are numerous examples of researchers producing inaccurate outcomes such as 'failing to report an outcome measure because it did not show any effect to presenting a biased review of the literature, focusing only on supportive evidence' (Stroebe and Hewstone 2013). In 2012, in medicine, one academic was found to have 193 published papers containing falsified research (Stroebe and Hewstone 2013).

It is important to realise that a *lack of evidence of efficacy* is not the same as *evidence of lack of efficacy* (Roth and Fonagy 2005). This means that if something has not been tested, there is no evidence that it doesn't work. The continuing disagreements over what constitutes evidence of efficacy and effectiveness have great importance when the NICE and SIGN guidelines are used as the basis for allocating funds for services and training in the NHS in the United Kingdom.

The results of this can be seen in the IAPT (Improving Access to Psychological Therapies) 2008–2011 service in England. Cognitive Behavioural Therapy demonstrated its efficacy in RCTs for a range of diagnosed mental illnesses including depression, anxiety and post-traumatic stress disorder. The government invested in setting up IAPT services to offer CBT to patients with a single diagnosis of either depression or anxiety. Training was provided for the delivery of both low- and high-intensity interventions. Analysis of the outcome data from people using IAPT services showed that counselling was as effective as CBT for people with depression. As a result some counselling was commissioned to be delivered in IAPT services. In the meantime many primary care counsellors have lost their jobs or re-trained to work in IAPT services.

Table 7.1 shows the powerful long-term impact of NICE guidelines on the primary care workforce delivering psychological therapy (Written Parliamentary answer to the question by Paul Burstow MP, former Care Services Minister, January 2013).

Professional and academic credibility and respect can lead to practical outcomes. Research that shows that counselling works, how it works and the cost effectiveness of counselling over other interventions can translate into jobs for counsellors. For example, an independent analysis of the outcomes for IAPT patients with depression showed that the outcomes for counselling were equivalent to the outcomes for Cognitive Behavioural Therapy (Glover, Webb et al. 2010). This resulted in the widening of approaches offered to IAPT clients to include counselling and to the commissioning of Counselling for Depression training for counsellors.

The use of randomised controlled trials of therapy has been criticised as unethical, as it leaves some clients on a waiting list, with no help. As waiting lists are the reality for many people seeking psychological therapy anyway, this objection does not carry much weight. A more valid query is whether the outcomes will transfer to everyday practice (Cooper and Reeves 2012).

Table 7.1   *Number of therapists by theoretical approach trained by the NHS 2008–2013*

Therapeutic intervention	2008–09	2009–10	2010–11	2011–12	2012–13	Total
CBT – low intensity	510	727	517	536	459	2,749
CBT for depression, anxiety & PTSD – high intensity	487	1,004	623	291	322	2,787
Counselling for depression – high intensity	0	0	64	68	132	264
Couples therapy for depression – high intensity	0	0	44	69	90	212
Brief Dynamic Therapy – high intensity	0	0	63	27	58	148
Interpersonal therapy – high intensity	0	0	86	62	155	323
Total	997	1,731	1,397	1,073	1,225	6,423

For example, a client in an RCT for depression will have a single diagnosis of depression. Counsellors argue that such a client is as rare as hen's teeth; most people will not be subject to the intense level of screening applied to RCT clients, and anyway no one would be refused counselling because they have multiple issues. In other words the working therapist has doubts about the transference to everyday practice of the findings of RCTs. The evidence from IAPT services suggests otherwise and that what works in a randomised controlled trial also works in an IAPT service. Others fear that the reliance on RCT evidence with its manuals of treatment will spread into everyday practice and damage the freedom to use clinical judgement and innovation.

Counselling and psychotherapy organisations are in a difficult position. If they continue to oppose the efficacy methodology of RCTs, then one approach, Cognitive Behavioural Therapy (CBT), will continue to dominate the efficacy evidence. If they attempt to set up and run RCTs on other approaches and techniques they may alienate many members. In addition, RCTs are very complex and expensive to set up and run. This makes it difficult for counselling and psychotherapy organisations to produce RCT evidence of the efficacy of their approach.

TYPES OF RESEARCH IN THE PSYCHOLOGICAL THERAPIES

The debate over the best methodology to evaluate the outcomes of psychological therapy has no clear answer and this book is not going to discover one. In this chapter I have divided research into the psychological therapies into three types: outcome studies, process studies and case studies.

Outcome research

Research question: Does it work? Outcome studies try to find out if the intervention has helped the client by looking at the difference in the client before and after therapy. Three types of factors have been related to outcome research in the psychological therapies: technique factors, participant/client factors and relationship factors, between the therapist and the client (Castonguay and Beutler 2006). Much recent outcome research in the United Kingdom has focused on technique factors of specific theoretical approaches for example, manualised treatment for post-traumatic stress disorder (PTSD) (Blisson, Shepherd et al. 2004).

Efficacy outcome research

Research question: Does this work? Efficacy outcome research is also described as evidence-based practice. This kind of research is often carried out in Randomised Controlled Trials (RCTs) and tests the efficacy of the technique, for example the use of CBT for irritable bowel syndrome (Lackner, Gudelski et al. 2010). A successful RCT will show that only the intervention can be responsible for the outcome/change in the clients in the trial, that no other factors could have had an effect. An RCT also tries to show that the outcome is achieved consistently in the clients in the trial. This is achieved by very detailed screening and selection of the clients in the trial and by the use of manualised theoretical interventions which all the therapists follow strictly. In this way the researchers try to eliminate every other factor that might influence the outcomes.

This type of research provides evidence that an intervention really works, as all other possible causes of change have been eliminated. If the trial is large, that is, it has a large number of patients with the same outcomes, this suggests that the approach will work in everyday life. That is, a large sample producing consistent evidence of efficacy will translate into effectiveness. It is difficult to have very large trials of counselling approaches, so this problem is addressed by pooling together several small trials of the same approach and analysing the results (meta-analysis). For example a meta-analysis of self-help versus face-to-face therapy for depression and anxiety found little difference in patient outcomes (Cuijpers, Donker et al. 2010).

One way of conducting RCTs in psychological therapies has been to randomly allocate some clients to the therapy and leave others on the waiting list. Another method is to test different theoretical approaches against each other and a non-therapy intervention and compare the outcomes. The 'placebo' or non-therapy is often usual, or GP care.

An RCT of geriatric patients with chronic depression found no difference in outcomes between counselling and usual care (Simpson, Corney et al. 2000). An RCT of non-directive counselling, cognitive behavioural therapy and usual general practitioner care in the management of depression found no significant difference in outcome between the two psychological therapies at 4 and 12 months. At both, patients in receipt of non-directive counselling were more satisfied. At 12 months there were no differences between all three groups (King, Sibbald et al. 2000).

Outcome trials of the efficacy of particular techniques can show the efficacy in a clinical trial and from this indicate that the techniques could potentially be useful in everyday practice. But, trial evidence does not prove the effectiveness of a technique in everyday practice.

Activity

Can you think of any other criticisms of this method of assessing the efficacy of counselling?

Can you think of any arguments to persuade counsellors to adopt this methodology?

Effectiveness outcome research

Research question: Does it work here? This research was carried out by the evaluation of actual everyday practice to see if the therapeutic intervention results in change in clients, and hopefully if it does, that the change is for the better and is the result of the therapeutic intervention, not just chance.

IAPT (Improving Access to Psychological Therapies) services use session-by-session measures, some for all clients, such as the Work and Social Adjustment Scale (WSAS) and others depending on the client's diagnosis. For depression there is the Patient Health Questionnaire (PHQ9) and for anxiety disorders the Generalised Anxiety Disorder Assessment (GAD7). These measures are used to assess severity and change. IAPT states that such session-by-session measurement improves both the quality and accountability of services (IAPT 2011, 2012). It is the case that the good outcomes achieved by counselling in IAPT services led to the commissioning of counselling alongside CBT.

One system widely used in the UK is CORE (Clinical Outcomes in Routine Evaluation), a routine outcome measuring system. CORE differs from Randomised Controlled Trials in two ways; it is not specific to any theoretical approach and assesses across a wide range of presenting issues. CORE evaluation therefore cannot be used to assess specific techniques in the same way as the outcomes of RCTs. CORE is used by counsellors in initial assessment, session-by-session monitoring and review sessions. CORE measures a client's level of psychological distress and changes to this. It measures client distress on common presenting issues such as anxiety, depression, trauma, physical problems, functioning, and risk of self-harm and the severity of the client's distress. The main CORE outcome measure contains 34 items, under four subheadings: wellbeing, symptoms, functioning and risk. Session-by-session use enables the counsellor and client to monitor and review progress or lack of it (www. coreims.co.uk).

CORE holds data on thousands of client sessions, in other words, it collects large-scale data outcomes from routine practice. The outcomes show that there is little or no difference between the theoretical approaches in terms of effectiveness; all show high levels of effectiveness.

One of the weaknesses of evaluation measures of effectiveness is that unless they are done every session, the effectiveness can appear to be more effective than may be the case. Every session evaluation enables counsellors to look back on the process and progress of clients who have unplanned endings, that is who do not turn up again. Outcome effectiveness research can also show the individual effectiveness of counsellors as not all counsellors are equally effective with clients.

There are other outcome evaluation tools. The Mental Health Recovery Star has ten areas for evaluation, each of which has a 'ladder of change', by which the client can monitor progress (www.mhpf.org.uk/resources/ publications). Overall, this kind of outcome research shows that on average there is improvement in the mental health and wellbeing of clients that lasts for one to two years after the therapy ends. A small percentage of clients get worse (5–10 per cent). These outcomes are comparable to drug treatments and have a higher compliance rate and appear to be cost effective.

Process research

Research question: How does it work?　This form of research is interested in effectiveness, but with a different focus to outcome studies. Process research searches for what is clinically important and meaningful, rather than measures of statistical significance. It looks at counsellor factors, client factors and the process of counselling in the everyday world of routine practice. The aim of process research is to identify the specific moments in therapy that bring about client change and through this to inform practice (Elliott 2010). Process research will look in fine detail at one session or a part of a single session. This is in marked contrast to the data collection of outcome research on effectiveness. Process research tends to involve active collaboration between the researcher and the counsellor and in some cases the client. The aim is to identify 'change events' in the therapy and then measure them. This research methodology can be traced back to the work of Carl Rogers on self-acceptance.

One form of process research was developed by Norman Kagan in the 1970s for use as a model for supervision; this is Interpersonal Process Recall (IPR) (1980). In this model therapy sessions are recorded then replayed by the supervisor with the counsellor or with both the counsellor and client. The aim is to help counsellors to become more aware of the dynamic of the counselling relationship by identifying material in counselling sessions that was unrecognised by both counsellor and client in the actual session but picked up during the IPR process. This is done by stopping the tape when, for example, the counsellor's verbal response seems incongruent with the non-verbal response. This attention to individual interactions has been developed into process outcome research which explores, for example, the effect of the depth of the counsellor's response on the client's own processing and outcomes. The findings show that counsellors' responses can both facilitate and halt the process for the client (Timulak 2010).

Case studies – counsellor and client

Research question: What worked or didn't work for you?   This section is subdivided into research on the counsellor and the client. Case studies have a long history in the psychological therapies, and remain one of the foundations of psychoanalytic training. Indeed, the psychoanalytic method in itself is seen as research and the source of psychoanalytic theory. One of the weaknesses of case study research is that the findings, although valid and credible, cannot be applied more generally (Yin 2003). While this is true, the findings of research into counsellors and clients do trigger thought and reflection in other counsellors, which in turn influences practice.

Counsellor-focused case study research   This research is qualitative and studies specific aspects of counsellors' experience or ways of working. It may be a study of a group of counsellors in relation to a specific question or issue which has implications for practice: for example, the impact of early attachment on clinical practice. It may be an auto-ethnographic study by a counsellor, in which the counsellor uses reflexivity to consciously embed him/herself in theory and practice and by so doing produce an auto-ethnography (Siddique 2011).

Research on therapeutic factors has tried to identify the personal characteristics of counsellors that contribute to positive client outcomes with mixed success. It appears that factors such as age, experience and continuing professional development do not correlate to client outcomes. However, effective counsellors seem to be able to effectively deal with client avoidance, have flexible interpersonal style and the ability to develop a strong therapeutic alliance (Laska, Smith et al. 2013).

Psychological therapists with a higher level of psychological wellbeing tend to have better outcomes. Counsellors who are given feedback on their client's progress seem to have better outcomes; this is also true where both counsellor and client are given feedback (Lambert, Harmon et al. 2005). This would seem to support session-by-session evaluation. The therapeutic relationship appears to be important to the counsellor as well as to the client. Research indicates that the therapeutic bond provides the counsellor with a high level of 'compassion satisfaction' which develops a vicarious resilience to traumatic client experience and vicarious traumatisation (Hunter 2012).

The researcher does not know at the start what the research will produce. Some research findings are uncomfortable. Counsellors seem to be poor at predicting the outcomes for clients, especially at the start of work with a client and if the relationship is weak (Worthen and Lambert 2007). Counsellors are also disinclined to take responsibility for the clients' early and unplanned ending of therapy, attributing such ending to the clients' circumstances rather than their own practice (Murdock, Edwards et al. 2010). There is little correspondence between what the counsellor identifies as significant in sessions and what the client identifies as significant (Elliot and Williams 2003; Castonguay and Beutler 2006; Dakin and Arean 2013). This leaves one counsellor, me, wondering about those 'aha!' moments I have had in sessions.

Findings from some meta-analyses suggest that counsellors are not all equally effective and it has been suggested that the variations between therapists have more impact than different theoretical approaches on the effectiveness of therapy (Wampold 2001). One research study found that 12 per cent of difference in client outcomes was due to the therapists (Laska, Smith et al. 2013). When asked to rate their own effectiveness, counsellors perceive themselves to be more effective than their peers (Lambert 2013). One piece of research into attitudes into the use of the internet in therapy found differences linked to the theoretical approach of the therapists, with psychoanalytic, psychodynamic and existential therapists less accepting of this medium of delivery (Perle, Langsam et al. 2013).

Client-focused case study research   Evidence from case study research is some-times seen as unable to contribute much to research on effectiveness, because it is difficult to take conclusions from individual cases and gener-alise these. Such case studies also do not follow such conventions as the random assignment of clients to therapists. Case study research on indi-vidual clients can be seen as the oldest form of research in Freud's case studies of his patients. Freud certainly generalised from particular cases. However, the psychoanalytic case study model is about the client, but it is not client-focused, in that the case study presents the analyst's experience, knowledge and perceptions of the client.

This section is about research on the client's experience in counselling which is often not the same as counsellors think clients experience. The ethical implications of conducting such research are discussed in Chapter 6. Several methods are used, for example questionnaires and the standard-ised evaluations used by IAPT psychological therapists. Such large-scale impersonal instruments provide data but lose the individual experience. More personal and intimate methods, such as interviews, have to be care-ful not to interfere in the therapeutic process, if carried out during the informant's therapy. This seems to be of more concern to counsellors than clients. Clients seem to respond positively to research, and gain from the self-reflection that comes in active participation. This is not surprising as active engagement in the process is welcomed by clients and is a well-established indicator of positive outcome (Cooper 2008; Bachelor 2013).

Another method is retrospective qualitative research on what the client found helpful and unhelpful. One study found that clients tend to see the relational and emotional aspects of significant moments as more impor-tant than cognitive aspects (Timulak 2007, 2010). Clients often attribute change to factors outside of the therapy rather than to the therapy itself. A reminder perhaps that while our therapeutic relationship is the only one we have with the client, he/she has many other relationships in their life.

One study found that clients saw the counsellor as someone who cared and in the early stages of therapy developed a dependence on the counsel-lor which later reduced by itself. These clients saw the therapy room as an expression of the counsellor's care. This generates thoughts about the control a counsellor has over the work environment and the potentially misleading messages clients may be receiving (Devlin and Nasar 2012).

Clients prefer a counsellor similar to themselves and clients' percep-tions of how the counsellor relates to them are significant for positive outcomes (Farsimadan, Draghi-Lorenz et al. 2007; Wampold and Budge 2012; Bachelor 2013). There are client factors that contribute to positive outcomes; for example, clients who have positive expectations, and are involved and motivated to change, do well especially if they are psychologically minded and have a high level of psychological functioning. Clients from low socio-economic groups find it more difficult to access and stay in psychological therapy (Kim and Cardemi 2012; Santiago, Kellman et al. 2013).

There have been many studies into what clients find helpful and unhelpful; the main findings and some references for further reading are given below. Clients like the basic relational skills of paraphrasing, listening and encouraging and empathy. They are less keen on questions, advice and frequent transference interpretations especially if things are not going well, when such interpretations are experienced as hostile.

Good outcomes seem to come from the client and counsellor working together towards agreed goals, when the counsellor can be open and honest about the process and rebuild the relationship if things have gone wrong. On the client side, good outcomes come from a motivation to change and a belief that the counsellor is a real person who cares. Clients do not seem to be as wedded to the one-to-one personal contact of the counselling room as counsellors. Many are happy to work in a range of media, such as phone, Skype, email and texting, all of which seem to be as effective as face-to-face work. In summary, research shows that the relationship is important for good outcomes whatever the medium of the therapy (Crist-Cristoph 2001; Anderson, Ogles et al. 2008; Castonguay, Boswell et al. 2010; McElvaney and Timulak 2013; Timulak and McElvaney 2013).

THE PLACE OF REFLECTIVE PRACTICE

Research and counsellor training

The first place that many counsellors come across research and research informed practice is during training. The nature of the research element in training courses varies depending on the course and the qualification it awards.

All university degree courses must include research at both undergraduate and postgraduate level. Any student taking a Masters degree will be required to produce a research-based dissertation, of probably between 15,000 and 20,000 words.

The specific requirements for counselling and psychotherapy degrees are set out below. Monitoring, evaluation and research is one of the seven core skills groups identified in the QAA subject benchmarks for degree programmes in counselling and psychotherapy at both degree and postgraduate levels.

All counsellors and psychotherapists need research skills that enable them to read and interpret research evidence related to practice. They also need to monitor and evaluate both individual practice and the work of a service or team. Routine outcome monitoring will involve the use of appropriate instruments that are subject to regular audit. Counsellors and psychotherapists may also engage in formal research in order to contribute to the developing knowledge and evidence base for their profession. (QAA 2013: 6)

In addition, for postgraduate qualifications counsellors are required to demonstrate the 'ability to successfully complete a substantial empirical research project, systematic review or systematic case study informed by wide current understandings in the discipline' (QAA 2013: 13). There are also higher level degrees, Professional Doctorates and PhDs which are research degrees.

Counselling training courses which deliver qualifications registered by Ofqual (Office of Qualifications and Examinations Regulation) tend to be at a lower level on the Qualification and Credit Framework and cannot award degrees. The time allocated to teaching about research varies in these courses. The Level 4 course delivered by one Awarding Organisation contains a module on research. This unit of 40 guided learning hours requires the student to understand the purpose of research, to know and evaluate research methodologies. In addition the student must carry out a piece of research using a selected methodology, present and critique both the findings and the methodology. It is therefore similar to the requirements of a university course. Other Awarding Organisation courses build research awareness into the other modules. The time given to research by private training courses varies.

BACP has a course accreditation scheme that accredits training courses that meet its standards across all three sectors. Research is included in two standards. One requires that students are taught about the research upon which the theoretical approach they are learning is based. The second is a separate criterion for research:

Students must be enabled to gain an awareness and working knowledge of research methodology to enable them to develop basic competences in small scale research projects. (BACP Course Accreditation Criterion B3.8)

Private training courses tend to do less direct teaching on research and research methodologies and lack the library facilities available at universities and colleges.

Career development

Many counsellors find their way into research later in their careers. Some through routine evaluation processes in everyday work, others through postgraduate degrees. Counsellors have many motivations for taking up research. It may be a way to achieve a promotion, part of agreed continuous professional development, a desire to gain a formal qualification, a personal goal, an interest in developing or creating new knowledge, or testing clinical experience with a formal methodology.

CONCLUSION

Strong arguments are made for all the psychological therapies to demonstrate both efficacy and effectiveness through research. While counselling needs to be research informed, research should take its place with the other elements that contribute to effective counselling: theory, supervision and clinical judgement (Cooper 2008).

Research findings cannot tell the counsellor what will happen with a specific client: the findings are either too general, as with outcome studies or too narrow, as with case studies. Research can help the counsellor think about what is happening and what may be a likely outcome. Sometimes sticking strictly to research findings can have negative results. For example, one study mentioned earlier indicates that clients like paraphrases and do not like questions. What if you have a client who opens up to questions and becomes irritated with paraphrases, saying if he wanted a parrot he'd buy one? Counsellors need to use clinical judgement as well as research findings in practice.

What counsellors can gain from being research informed is the habit of critical reflection on both the research findings and the application of these to practice. For most people this will be the extent of the engagement with research. Others will become more immersed and perhaps add new knowledge to the field.

There is so much more research to be done to find answers to Gordon Paul's 1967 questions, with which this chapter began: '*What* treatment, by *whom,* is most effective for *this* individual with *that* specific problem, and under *which* set of circumstances?'

REFERENCES

Anderson, T., B. M. Ogles, et al. (2008). 'Therapist effects: facilitative interpersonal skills as a predictor of therapist sucess.' *Journal of Clinical Psychology* **65**(7): 755–68.

Bachelor, A. (2013). 'Clients' and therapists' views of the therapeutic alliance: similarities, differences and relationship to therapy outcomes.' *Clinical Psychoogy and Psychotherapy* **20**(2): 118–35.

Bager-Charleson, S. (2010). *Reflective Practice in Counselling and Psychotherapy*. Poole, Learning Matters.

Blisson, J. C., J. P. Shepherd, et al. (2004). 'Early cognitive behavioural therapy for post-traumatic stress symptoms after physicial injury: Randomized controlled trial.' *British Journal of Psychiatry* **184**: 63–9.

Castonguay, L. G. and L. E. Beutler (2006). 'Principles of therapeutic change: a taskforce on participants, relationships and technical factors.' *Journal of Clinical Psychology* **62**(6): 631–8.

Castonguay, L. G., J. F. Boswell, et al. (2010). 'Training implications on harmful effects of psychological treatments.' *American Psychologist* **65**(1): 34–9.

Cooper, M. (2008). *Essential Research Findings in Counselling and Psychotherapy*. London, SAGE/ BACP.

Cooper, M. and A. Reeves (2012). 'The role of randomised controlled trials in developing an evidence-base for counselling.' *Counselling and Psychotherapy Research* **12**(4): 303–7.

Crist-Cristoph, P. (2001). 'Therapist–patient relationship.' *International Encyclopedia of the Social and Behavioural Sciences*: 15662–5.

Cuijpers, P., T. Donker, et al. (2010). 'Is guided self-help as effective as face-to-face psychotherapy for depression and anxiety disorders? A systematic review and meta-analysis of comparative outcome studies.' *Psychological Medicine* **40**(12): 1943–57.

Dakin, E. K. and P. Arean (2013). 'Patient perspectives on the benefits of psychotherapy for late life depression.' *American Journal of Geriatric Psychiatry* **21**(2): 155–63.

Devlin, A. S. and J. L. Nasar (2012). 'Impressions of psychotherapists' offices: do therapists and clients agree?' *Professional Psychology Research and Practice* **43**(2): 118–22.

Elliot, M. and D. Williams (2003). 'The client experience of counselling and psychotherapy.' *Counselling Psychology Review* **18**(1): 34.

Elliott, R. (2010). 'Psychotherapy change process research: realizing the promise.' *Psychotherapy Research* **20**(2): 123–35.

Etherington, K. (2004). *Becoming a Reflexive Researcher: Using Ourselves in Research*. London, Jessica Kingsley.

Farsimadan, F., R. Draghi-Lorenz, et al. (2007). 'Process and outcome of therapy in ethnically similar and dissimilar therapeutic dyads.' *Psychotherapy Research* **17**(5): 567–75.

Glover, G., M. Webb and F. Evison (2010). *Improving Access to Psychological Therapies. A Review of the Progress made by Sites in the First Roll-out Year*. North East Public Health Observatory.

Hunter, S. V. (2012). 'Walking in the sacred spaces in the therapist bond: therapists's experience of compassion satisfaction coupled with the potential for vicarious traumatisation.' *Family Process* **51**(2): 179–202.

IAPT (2011). *The IAPT Data Handbook. Guidance on Recording and Monitoring Outcomes to Support Local Evidence-based Practice.* Version 2.0. London, Department of Health.

IAPT (2012). *IAPT 3 Year Report. The First Million Patients.* London, Department of Health.

Kagan, N. (1980). 'Influencing human interaction – Eighteen years with IPR.' In A. K. Hess (Ed.), *Psychotherapy Supervision: Theory, Research and Practice.* New York, Wiley: 262–83.

Kim, S. and K. Cardemi (2012). 'Effective psychotherapy with low income clients: the importance of attending to social class.' *Journal of Contemporary Psychotherapy* **42**(1): 27–35.

King, M., B. Sibbald, et al. (2000). 'Randomised controlled trial of non-directive counselling, cognitive-behaviour therapy and usual general practitioner care in the management of depression as well as mixed anxiety and depression in primary care.' *Health Technology Assessment* **4**(19): 1–83.

Lackner, J. M., G. D. Gudelski, et al. (2010). 'Rapid response to Cognitive Behaviour Therapy for Irritable Bowel Syndrome.' *Clinical Gastroenterology and Hepatology* **8**: 426–32.

Lambert, M. J. (2013). *Keynote Address.* BACP Research Conference, Coventry, BACP.

Lambert, M. J., C. Harmon, et al. (2005). 'Providing feedback to psycho-therapists on their patients' progress: clinical results and practice suggestions.' *Journal of Clinical Psychology* **61**(2): 165–74.

Laska, K. M., T. L. Smith, et al. (2013). 'Uniformity of evidence-based treatments in practice? Therapist effects in the delivery of cognitive processing therapy for PTSD.' *Journal of Counselling Psychology* **60**(1): 31–41.

McElvaney, J. and L. Timulak (2013). 'Clients' experience of therapy and its outcomes in "good" and "poor" outcome psychological therapy in a primary care setting: an exploratory study.' *Counselling and Psychotherapy Research.* iFirst online publication pp. 1–8. DOI 10.1080/14733145.2012.761258

Murdock, N. L., C. Edwards and T. B. Murdock (2010). 'Therapists' attributions for clients' premature termination. Are they self-serving?' *Psychotherapy Theory, Research, Practice, Training* **47**(2): 221–34.

Perle, J. G., L. C. Langsam, A. Randell, S. Lutchman, A. B. Levine, A. P. Odland, B. Nierneberg and C. D. Marker (2013). 'Current and future clinical psychologists' opinions of internet-based interventions.' *Journal of Clinical Psychology* **69**(1): 100–13.

QAA (2013). *Subject benchmark Statement. Counselling and Psychotherapy.* Gloucester, Quality Assurance Agency for Higher Education.

Roth, A. and P. Fonagy (2005). *What Works for Whom? A Critical Review of Psychotherapy Research.* New York, The Guilford Press.

Santiago, C. D., S. Kellman, et al. (2013). 'Poverty and mental health. How do low-income adults and children fare in psychotherapy?' *Journal of Clinical Psychology* **69**(2): 115–26.

Schon, D. A. (1983). *The Reflective Practitioner: How Professionals Think in Action*. London, Maurice Temple Smith.

Siddique, S. (2011). 'Being in-between: The relevance of ethnography and auto-ethnography for psychotherapy research.' *Counselling and Psychotherapy Research* **11**(4): 310–16.

Simpson, S., R. Corney, et al. (2000). 'A randomized controlled trial to evaluate the effectiveness and cost-effectiveness of counselling patients with chronic depression.' *Health Technology Assessment* **4**(36): 36–83.

Stroebe, W. and M. Hewstone (2013). 'Primed, but not suspect.' *Times Higher Education* **2090**: 34–9.

Timulak, L. (2007). 'Identifying core categories of client-identified impact of helpful events in psychotherapy: a qualitative meta-analysis.' *Psychotherapy Research* **17**(3): 305–14.

Timulak, L. (2010). 'Significant events in psychotherapy: an update of research findings, client identified important moments.' *Psychology and Psychotherapy* **83**(4): 421–47.

Timulak, L. and J. McElvaney (2013). 'Qualitative meta-analysis of insight events in psychotherapy.' *Counselling Psychology Quarterly* **26**(2): 131–50.

Wampold, B. E. and S. Budge (2012). 'The relationship – and its relationship to the common and specific factors in psychotherapy.' *The Counseling Psychologist* **40**(4): 601–23.

Wampold, B. E. (2001). *The Great Psychotherapy Debate: Models, Methods and Findings*. Mahwah, NJ, Erlbaum.

Watson, J. C. and D. L. Rennie (1994). 'Qualitative analysis of clients' subjective experience of significant moments during the exploration of problematic reactions.' *Journal of Counselling Psychology* **41**(4): 500–9.

Worthen, V. E. and M. J. Lambert (2007). 'Outcome oriented supervision: advantages of adding systematic client tracking to supportive consultations.' *Counselling and Psychotherapy Research* **7**(1): 48–53.

Yin, R. K. (2003). *Case Study Research, Design and Methods*. Thousand Oaks, CA, Sage.

8 THE STRUCTURE OF THE PROFESSION AND CAREERS IN COUNSELLING

This chapter outlines the structure of the profession and covers some of the areas of counselling missing so far, namely the professional associations for counselling, supervision and career development opportunities for counsellors. It gives a snapshot of working counsellors. Finally it looks at the practical aspect of employment, what jobs are available and most importantly what they pay.

This book began with a chapter on What is counselling? – and found it difficult to come up with a clear succinct answer. This should not be so surprising as counselling began as an undefined activity, claimed and delivered by a wide range of people. In 1977 counsellors included:

People who recognise a counselling component in their work – clergy, doctors, nurses, lawyers, professionals and voluntary workers.

Teachers and others appointed into schools to spend most of the time counselling. Those who work in careers guidance.

Marriage counsellors, bereavement, youth and pastoral counsellors. (SCAC 1977: 8)

Only the last group would be described as counsellors today, and that group has expanded from face-to-face work to develop the relational skills needed to counsel in virtual worlds.

There have been incremental changes over the years, moving counselling towards recognition as a profession. Similarly, there seems to be a widespread understanding of the difference between counselling and advice and guidance. National standards for training have been set in the QAA Benchmark statement for counselling and psychotherapy and the lower level qualifications on the QCF and SCQF and there are counsellor job descriptions in the NHS Agenda for Change. There are still groups who oppose the professionalisation of counselling in any form. House and Totton, two such opponents, wrote in 1997 that the founders of counselling and psychotherapy 'thought what they had created was "wild, extraordinary and unsuitable for domestication"' (1997: 5). Counselling can be all of those things, but also needs an ethical awareness and accountability to clients. These latter are two of the elements of a profession.

A list of the elements that constitute a profession also forms some of the topics of the chapters of this book: training, personal development, theoretical approaches, the establishment of a boundary with counselling skills, ethics and research (Aldridge 2010).

There are many organisations representing the psychological therapies, and these differ in size and purpose. Twenty-nine organisations that registered counsellors and psychotherapists were identified when mapping the field for the Department of Health in 2005 (Aldridge and Pollard 2005). Figure 8.1 shows the relative size of the five largest associations in 2012.

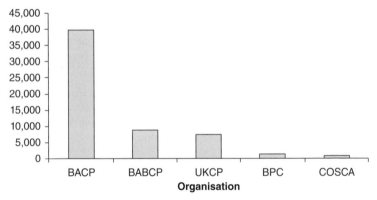

Figure 8.1   *The membership numbers of the major professional associations for counselling and psychotherapy (BACP 2013)*

As the figure shows, BACP is by far the largest professional association for counselling and psychotherapy in the United Kingdom. One of the reasons for BACP's size, is that membership is not restricted to any particular theoretical approach or work context.

Much of the information in this chapter is derived from BACP sources as the large numbers from which it is drawn enables it to be used as a proxy for counselling in the United Kingdom. It is estimated that there are between 60,000 and 100,000 people practising counselling in the United Kingdom today (Mann 2006; Symons 2012). Many counsellors belong to more than one professional association.

The organisations and professional associations in counselling take several forms and deliver different functions. BACP's membership criteria are not based on any particular theoretical approach or work setting. It is therefore an umbrella organisation and accredits courses, services and individuals to generic rather than specialist standards. Some professional associations represent defined or specialist areas and membership is restricted to counsellors within the work context, for example, Relate, the Federation of Drug and Alcohol Professionals, Counsellors and Psychotherapists in Primary Care and the Association of Christian Counsellors. These organisations may approve or accredit both training courses and individuals practising in the specialist area. Others are organisations for specific theoretical approaches, for example the British Association for the Person-Centred Approach. Both of these types of organisations are small, because they are by definition self-limiting. Another form of organisation is one that has close links with training courses, for example the Human Givens Institute and Human Givens training and the National Counselling Society and Chrysalis Courses.

Counselling professional associations usually have grades of membership for people who wish to work as a counsellor; some also have grades for people who are interested but not practitioners. A usual pattern would be to join as a student, then when qualified move to become a full registrant or member and later enter higher grades of membership. These higher grades are often called 'accredited' and call for the assessment and quality assurance of practice. Training courses often encourage students to join a professional organisation to give them a sense of belonging and provide them with ethical and practice guidelines for placements.

Activity

Using the internet/Google, find and read the websites of a range of professional organisations for counselling. Compare the information, for example, on intended members, fees, membership benefits, ethical codes and professional conduct processes.

What factors would influence you to join a professional association?

(Continued)

(Continued)

Table 8.1 *Features of professional associations*

	British Association for Counselling and Psychotherapy (BACP)	British Association for Behavioural and Cognitive Psychotherapies (BABCP)	United Kingdom Council for Psychotherapy (UKCP)	British Psychoanalytic Council (BCP)	Counselling and Psychotherapy in Scotland (COSCA)
Membership grades					
Fees for membership					
Journal for members					
CPD events for members					
Ethical framework					
Professional Conduct procedure					
Marketing					
Professional credibility					
Information and guidance					
AVR accreditation					

There are also commercial organisations in the counselling field. In Chapter 3 on training, the Registered Awarding Organisations were mentioned. These are organisations that develop qualifications to be approved by Ofqual (the Office of Qualifications and Examination Regulation) and placed on the QCF (Qualifications and Credit Framework) and the Scottish equivalent, the SCQF (Scottish Credit and Qualification Framework). The qualifications are delivered in centres approved and overseen by the Registered Awarding Organisation. Most deliver a wide range of subjects, but one, the Counselling and Psychotherapy Central Awarding Body (CPCAB) delivers only counselling and psychotherapy qualifications. There are also commercial directories that advertise counsellors; some, like Thompsons and Yellow Pages are generic, and there are also specialist ones for counselling like the Counselling Directory and Counselling Ltd that advertise and promote the counsellors on their lists.

ACCREDITED VOLUNTARY REGISTERS

The change of government policy on professional regulation in 2010, mentioned in Chapter 1, introduced a new quality assurance scheme for counsellors as well as all unregulated health and social care professions, the Accreditation of Voluntary Registers (AVR) scheme, operated by the Professional Standards Authority for Health and Social Care. This scheme, made law in the 2012 Health and Social Care Act, is described in the Act as follows:

25G Power of the Authority to accredit voluntary registers

(1) Where a regulatory body or other person maintains a voluntary register, the Authority may, on an application by the body or other person, take such steps as it considers appropriate for the purpose of establishing whether the register meets such criteria as the Authority may from time to time set ('accreditation criteria').

(2) Accreditation criteria may, in particular, relate to—

   (a) the provision to the Authority of information in connection with the establishment, operation or maintenance of register;

   (b) publication of the names of persons included in the register or who have been removed from the register (whether voluntarily or otherwise);

   (c) the establishment or operation of a procedure for appeals from decisions relating to inclusion in or removal from the register.

(3) If the Authority is satisfied that a voluntary register meets the accreditation criteria, it may accredit the register.

(4) The Authority may carry out periodic reviews of the operation of registers accredited under this section for the purpose of establishing whether they continue to meet the accreditation criteria.

The central function of the scheme is to promote the interests of service users and members of the public and to promote best practice and good governance in the performance of voluntary registration functions (Department of Health 2012, Part 7, Sections 228–9).

The original move in 2007 to statutorily regulate counselling and psychotherapy met with fierce opposition from some within the field, leading to an application for a judicial review against the Health Professions Council. In contrast, the introduction of the AVR scheme has received a positive welcome, as it does not seek to homogenise counselling and psychotherapy. The purpose is the same, to protect the public and the service user from poor or bad practice, but the philosophical basis in Right Touch Regulation fits better with the values of counselling (www.professional-standards.org.uk/policy-and-research/right-touch-regulation).

In AVR scheme, the organisation that holds the register must demonstrate that it meets all the standards and provide evidence of how the standard has been met. For the first time, any counselling organisation making an application for the accreditation of its register will be subject to objective external scrutiny. Some of the things that may be taken for granted within an organisation look very different to external eyes!

Some counsellors were disappointed when it became clear that counselling would not be subject to statutory regulation because they saw statutory regulation as conferring government recognition and status on counselling. The purpose of the AVR scheme is to provide the public and employers with a mark of quality, not a mark of status for the professionals on the register. It can be argued that voluntarily undertaken regulation will lead to fewer instances on poor or bad practice, because the individual has the responsibility to monitor his/her practice, rather than devolving this to a regulatory council. This is the view taken by the Professional Standards Authority in its Accreditation of Voluntary Registers scheme.

The intention is that employers and commissioners and members of the public will be advised to only use someone displaying the AVR logo, that is, only people who are registered on an Accredited Voluntary Register. It is hoped that in the fields of health and social care this will become as well known as the 'Corgi' mark for gas fitters was. At present BACP and the National Counselling Society are the only accredited voluntary register for the psychological therapies (www.bacpregister.org.uk/). (Psychiatrists and clinical and counselling psychologists are already subject to statutory regulation.)

In this scheme it is the register, not the registrant that is accredited, and the accredited register holds the responsibility for the conduct of its registrants. Registrants on accredited registers can use the AVR logo to advertise that they are on an accredited register.

THE STRUCTURE OF COUNSELLING

Like most professions, counsellors are expected to undertake continuing professional development (CPD) throughout their careers. This can take many forms, the best known is supervision, although this is often seen as separate from continuing professional development. One of the features that marks counselling out from most other professions in the United Kingdom is the requirement for supervision of practice throughout working life (Wheeler and Richards 2007; Scaife 2009). This is also a major difference between counsellors in the United Kingdom and Europe and counsellors in the USA.

It is common in some professions for a form of mentoring and supervision to be obligatory during training and in the early years of practice. There is a form of 'provisional licence' for teachers in England in 'Newly Qualified Teacher' (NQT) status, and requirements to be met to move to full qualified status. For counsellors in the United Kingdom supervision is an ethical requirement throughout practice (Bond 2010). Supervision 'is a formal relationship in which there is a contractual agreement that the therapist will present their work with clients in an open and honest way that enables the supervisor to have insight into the way in which the work was conducted' (Wheeler and Richards 2007: 4). There are different models of supervision, but all include clarity about roles, relationships and the responsibilities of the supervisor.

It is suggested that counsellors probably need different sorts of supervision during their careers, with more guidance and an educational focus for students and more self-reflection later in a career. Supervision can be one-to-one or in a group; students tend to feel safer in one-to-one supervision but lose the opportunity to learn from other people's experience. Group supervision is common with a supervisor facilitating the group in training and early in the career, but often shifting to peer group supervision with experienced counsellors. Professional associations like BACP may specify the amount of supervision required for certain grades of members, for example 1.5 hours a month for accredited counsellors.

Counsellors' requirement for supervision has caused misunderstanding about the capacity of counsellors to work autonomously, as the term 'supervision' is often understood to mean managerial oversight and direct responsibility for clinical work of the supervisee. In other words, a counsellor's need for supervision is evidence of immature or lower level work than an independent practitioner. Other terms have been suggested to solve this, consultative support being one. But to date, nothing has proved popular, so counsellors are stuck with explaining what counselling supervision means.

Supervision is seen as one of the foundations and unique features of counselling. It is seen as essential for the maintenance of standards of practice. This has been accepted by employers, who build supervision into employment contracts. Supervision can also be used in the sanctions imposed when a complaint has been upheld in a professional conduct case. A supervisor may be appointed to assist the counsellor to reflect on the sanctions, learn from them and undertake activities to improve practice.

The BACP *Ethical Framework for Good Practice in Counselling and Psychotherapy* states 'All counsellors, psychotherapists, trainers and supervisors are required to have regular and on-going formal supervision/consultative support for their work, in accordance with professional requirements' (BACP 2010) There is an assumption that supervision 'is a good thing': that it improves the effectiveness of the practice of the counsellor, or that clients have a better experience and better outcomes as a result of supervision. To date, there is very limited research evidence to support any of these assumptions. There is tentative evidence that supervisees incorporate the learning from supervision into practice and that the perceived trustworthiness of the supervisor is a factor in effective supervision (Wheeler and Richards 2007). To date most of the research has been carried out on supervisees in training in the USA. This presents a dilemma; supervision is so embedded in counselling training and practice that it would be very difficult to abandon it on the research evidence presented so far, and no one has proposed this. This suggests that counsellors find supervision a positive experience and believe that it supports practice and safeguards clients. Is it the case that a lack of evidence is not in itself evidence of a lack of effectiveness? Or is supervision an article of faith for counsellors?

THE COUNSELLING WORKFORCE

Counselling has been and remains a second profession for many people and this is clear from the age profiles of counsellors. Over 80 per cent of counsellors are women, and this proportion has changed little since the 1980s (Aldridge 2010). Various reasons have been suggested for this: that women are socialised to enter caring professions; that the part-time nature of training and practice suits women more than men. These arguments smack of patriarchal attitudes, but whatever the reason, counselling is a female middle-aged occupation. This of course may be a self-perpetuating pattern, as many clients are middle-aged women. Perhaps the options are to become a client or a counsellor!

There are also few counsellors from minority ethnic groups and lower socio-economic groups (BACP 2012). Yet the evidence shows that many clients prefer counsellors with similar backgrounds to their own (Farsimadan, Draghi-Lorenz et al. 2007; BACP 2012; McLaughlin, Holliday et al. 2013). There is an element of common sense in the fact that a grieving widower in his 80s may find it difficult to build a therapeutic alliance with a 20-something counsellor, and a 17-year-old may struggle to confide in someone who reminds him of his gran. The United Kingdom is a multi-cultural society but the psychological therapies do not seem to have developed in parallel to understand and work with client needs arising from this (Moodley 2007). There is a clear need for both younger counsellors and counsellors from a wider socio-economic span.

Many counsellors have already been working in a helping profession before entering counselling, for example one counsellor, now working in a University counselling service recalled:

> After my degree, I trained as a social worker, and then worked in a variety of settings, elderly residential care, youth work and voluntary sector projects before moving into counselling. Because I didn't settle in any of these, to me counselling feels like my first profession.

But others see counselling as a second profession: 'I was a successful businessman running my own building company and I wanted to give something back. I started as a volunteer with the Samaritans, then wanted to know more so did a counselling training.'

One consequence of this is that counsellors tend to be middle-aged, over two-thirds between the ages of 40 and 60. Despite the introduction of undergraduate degrees in counselling, this age profile has changed little. Although people enter counselling at a later age than most professions, counsellors also seem to continue working later in life beyond the statutory retirement age. It is known that many counsellors start in voluntary work and perhaps after a few years, still without paid employment some people give up. It may be that this is the sort of time it takes to accumulate enough practice to gain accreditation. For example for BACP accreditation counsellors can take up to six years gaining practice. If having achieved accreditation, there is still no or little paid employment, again counsellors may give up. It is a fact that there are fewer counsellors in practice than would be expected from the number who qualify each year.

The geographic spread of counsellors is generally proportionate with that of the general population spread: over 80 per cent of the UK population and over 80 per cent of counsellors live in London and the South East.

There are proportionally more counsellors in Northern Ireland than in England, Scotland and Wales. Perhaps this is the result of the recent history of the Troubles and a more publicly recognised need for psychological help as evidenced in the funding of the Victims and Survivors Service by the Office of the First Minister.

CAREERS IN COUNSELLING

There are several career paths open to counsellors as shown in Figure 8.2. This section looks at each of these in turn, starting with the role of counsellor.

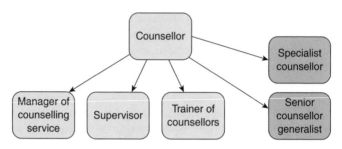

Figure 8.2   *Careers for counsellors*

The counsellor

The first task for a newly qualified counsellor is to find clients. Counsellors who have trained while working, for example, as a nurse or teacher often find it frustrating that they are unable to practise as counsellors in that role. It can feel as if all the training has been for nothing, when on return to the previous role they are not recognised as counsellors. This is made worse if the clinical placement was in their place of employment. A few newly qualified counsellors will be retained by their placement agency, but these are few and there is a queue of students seeking placements snapping at their heels. It is quite common for counsellors to work in a voluntary capacity while seeking paid employment and/or building up hours to be eligible to apply for professional accreditation. Some agencies advertise for such voluntary counsellors – see the MIND advertisement below (p. 178).

It is not unethical or selfish to want to be paid for the work you do. It just seems quite difficult to find counselling jobs that provide a living wage. Various surveys have found that counsellors tend to work part time, for between 5 and 20 hours a week and see clients on average for between 6 and 10 sessions. What isn't known is whether this part-time work and short-term counselling is by counsellor choice. A survey of BACP counsellors in Northern Ireland found some counselling was terminated because the allocated number of sessions had been reached, regardless of the client's progress (Aldridge, Coulter and Robinson 2012). Many of the jobs described later on in this chapter are part time, indicating that this is employer choice. BACP recommends that counsellors should do no more than 20 hours a week direct client work; however, it is difficult to know if this is held to in practice.

There are conflicting demands at play within counselling. Students need placements to complete an amount of supervised practice in order to qualify. Qualified counsellors need supervised practice hours to become eligible for accreditation with professional associations. As a result both groups deliver voluntary counselling and as a result deny counsellors paid employment. One possible reason for the low salaries on offer is that it is easy to find counsellors who will work voluntarily. That is, training courses and professional associations suppress the market for paid employment. In other health related professions things are different; clinical experience built into the qualification and placement providers are paid in the case of physiotherapy. Nurses have access to NHS student bursaries and the training is 50 per cent theory at a University and 50 per cent practice in the NHS.

Many counsellors 'portfolio' work, that is they counsel in several different settings and for various employers. It is quite common for counsellors to have contracts with several Employment Assistance Providers (EAPs) as this maximises the potential clients. It seems that the longer someone stays in counselling the greater proportion of their income derives from counselling. It could also be that people give up and leave counselling altogether if they cannot find enough paid work, thus leaving the work to be shared among a smaller number.

I trained in a group of 14; two years after qualification two of us were employed as counsellors and three were doing some counselling but not in employment. After five years, I was the only one left.

Counsellors work as employees in the public sector such as the Health service, education and prisons, and for agencies in the commercial and voluntary sector. EAPS also offer work, mainly in the form of contracted affiliates, often for telephone counselling. This means that the counsellor is on the EAPS list, but it does not guarantee clients. Counsellors also work in a voluntary capacity; this used to be limited to the voluntary sector but such things as 'honorary therapists' are appearing in the public sector.

Between a third and a half of counsellors supplement their income by private practice charging on average between £30 and £50 per hour (AGCAS 2012). This covers a range of fees from £30 per session to £120.

There are several differences between employment and private practice. Some are given below. In theory a counsellor in private practice has a choice over which clients to see. She does not have to record routine outcome measures on private clients. This does not imply that counsellors in private practice are unconcerned about clients' progress. They may have their own outcome measures, but they will not be linked into such data bases as the IAPT minimum data set which collects and analyses the outcomes and performance of all IAPT services in England. Private practice, especially if working from home can be very isolating and it can be difficult to 'leave the client in the consulting room'. The counsellor in private practice will have to carry out initial assessments that are often done by someone else in an agency. She will also have set up an efficient financial system, including asking for payment.

Activity

What other differences might there be between working in each of the settings set out in Table 8.2?

Table 8.2   *Differences between work contexts*

Employment context	Features
Employed by the NHS	
Employed by a small charitable agency	
Work as a member of a group of counsellors taking paying and free clients	
Working in private practice from a rented consulting room	
Working in private practice from home	

The 2005 survey found that only 13 per cent of counsellors employed in the Health Service held a qualification from a private provider compared to 51 per cent who had a University qualification. This might suggest that NHS employers prefer to employ counsellors with University qualifications. Counsellors work in all sectors, and the public/private split is becoming less important. The theoretical approach has become more important in the Health Service with the development of NICE

Table 8.3 *Agenda for Change Pay rates from 1 April 2013*

Band 4	£18,838–£22,016
Band 5	£21,388–£27,901
Band 6	£25,783–£34,530
Band 7	£30,764–£40,558
Band 8a	£39,239–£47,088

Guidelines on common mental health conditions such as anxiety and depression. In the first three years the Improving Access to Psychological Therapies programme delivered only Cognitive Behavioural Therapy to patients with mild to moderate depression and anxiety. The programme has now been expanded to include humanistic counselling for depression, brief dynamic therapy, interpersonal therapy and behavioural couples therapy. All of these require additional approved training and most of the High Intensity jobs in IAPT are taken by clinical psychologists.

Counsellors working in the NHS include primary care and specialists such as oncology and genetic counsellors (www.nhscareers.nhs.uk/explain-by-career/psychological therapies). As NHS employees, counsellors are included in Agenda for Change, the national agreement on pay and conditions of service for NHS staff other than medical staff and very senior managers. Counsellors have job descriptions at salary bands 5–8, but counsellors have been employed on Band 4 (see Table 8.3).

The changes in the NHS taking place at the moment mean that it is difficult to predict the job market for counsellors. The introduction of the IAPT programme in England resulted in a reduction in the number of primary care counsellors based in GP surgeries. The introduction of GP Commissioning Consortia may result in further changes in the provision of the psychological therapies.

Other changes to the delivery of the health service may also have an impact on employment. The psychological therapies are one of the services in which the Any Qualified Provider scheme has been piloted. This scheme allows any service or individual to apply to be recognised as a 'Qualified Provider of a specified service'. A GP will then give the patient the information about which qualified providers there are for the service he/she needs and the patient makes the choice. Some counselling services and counsellors have become Qualified Providers on the national list. This blurs the distinction between the public and private centre with charitable organisations like Relate and Mind becoming qualified providers and being paid by the NHS to deliver what to all intents and purposes are NHS services. Like EAP contracts, there is no guarantee of clients. In Northern

Ireland, the government is in the process of investing in the expansion of counselling in both the secondary and primary care sector.

Counsellors who specialise

One career path is to specialise with a particular client group, for example eating disorders, autism, children and young people and many more.

Work with children and young people is an area of growth for counselling. Northern Ireland and Wales are committed to support counselling in schools. The Welsh government has a policy of a counsellor in every secondary school which will be expanded to primary schools (Department for Children, Education, Lifelong Learning and Skills 2008). Northern Ireland has provided an independent counselling service in schools since 2006 (Department of Education 2012). England lags behind and at present school counselling is provided by organisations such as the Place2Be, although some schools, especially private schools, employ counsellors. One such role is advertised later in this chapter.

One counsellor began as a social worker and specialised in working with families from the BSL (British Sign Language) community. She realised that many of the emotional and mental health needs of BSL users were not being met. She trained as a counsellor and used her combined skills to develop a counselling service for BSL users.

Voluntary sector agencies represent one of the largest employment sectors for counsellors, but as some of the advertisements below show, these are not always paid employment. Such agencies do offer career progression into supervision and management.

Supervision

A natural career progression is from counselling into supervision, often combining the two. As long as there are counsellors there will be the need for supervisors, but supervision is usually monthly, so a supervision practice will need to be large to produce the equivalent income to weekly counselling. Supervisors are required to have supervision for their own supervision work. This gives rise to the question of where does it all end, or is it infinite, like a never ending set of Russian dolls? It has been described as a job creation scheme for counsellors.

It is common for supervisors to have multiple relationships and responsibilities, some of which are shown in Figure 8.3.

A supervisor will have a range of responsibilities, depending on the context in which the supervisee works. Supervisors of trainees in clinical placements will be asked to evaluate and write reports on the competence of the trainees and to ensure that the trainee does not exceed the limits of

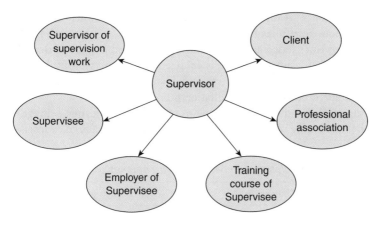

Figure 8.3 *The responsibilities of the supervisor*

his/her competence. It is normal for a trainee to have a supervisor from the same theoretical orientation as the training course, to assist with the translation of theory into practice. This supervision will have educative and mentoring elements, especially if the supervisor works in the placement agency. Some supervisors will provide in-house supervision to colleague counsellors employed in an agency and this can give rise to challenging situations if the supervisor believes that client safety is being compromised by poor practice.

Some professional associations, for example BACP, strongly advocate that counsellors should have a supervisor independent of their employment, in order to remove anxieties about the possible conflicts of interest. For the same reasons, a supervisor should not be a counsellor's line manager.

Whatever the relationship between supervisor, counsellor and employer, the supervision contract should cover what actions will be taken by the supervisor if he/she considers the supervisee to be working beyond their competence or behaving in an unethical way that places clients at risk. In effect this means that the supervisor is evaluating the supervisee's practice. In a situation where a supervisee ignores or denies the issues that have arisen in supervision and continues working in a particular way or with a particular client, a supervisor has two options. First, if the counsellor is employed, an approach can be made to the employer; second, and not mutually exclusive, the supervisor can raise a complaint with the supervisee's professional association. In both cases, the supervisee would need to know in advance.

A counsellor working towards professional body accreditation will need the supervisor to present such an evaluation or affirmation of client work presented. It is not unusual for a supervisor to advise the supervisee that he/she is not yet ready to apply for accreditation and refuse to support the application. Hurtful as this may be to the supervisee, it is worth trusting the supervisor's judgement, as he/she will be a good judge, and doubtless have had many supervisees apply for accreditation previously. A natural reaction can be to change supervisor, but such a change will be picked up and explored during the accreditation process.

Supervision can be in both a one-to-one and group format, with group supervision more cost effective for employers. For experienced counsellors,

Table 8.4 *Examples of supervision training courses*

Sector	University	QCF	Private
Qualification level	Postgraduate certificate	Level 6 diploma	Institution's own certificate and diploma
Duration of course	1 year part time	90 guided learning hours	Certificate: 52 hours face-to-face Diploma: 6 days
Entry requirements	Minimum 3 years post-qualifying experience Member of a professional body Must have in place before start of course supervision of 2 counsellors for a minimum of 6 months	Diploma in counselling and substantial experience	Minimum 3 years post-qualifying experience. Certificate: already supervising (or wish to) Diploma: already supervising and had some supervision training
Practicum requirements	12 hours of supervision of counsellors 8 hours of supervision for own supervision	15 hours a week of supervision 5 hours of supervision of supervision	Certificate: none Diploma: 20 hours of supervised supervision
Course content	Learning styles, models of supervision, intervention strategies, group supervision, evaluation and assessment	Professional framework, key skills, relationships, use of self, theory and research in supervision	Definition, relationships, models, key skills and structure. Ethical framework. Contracts & issue of diversity & equality
Fee	£1,750	£249	Certificate: £950 Diploma: £1,050

group supervision, with group members taking it in turn to act as facilitator can be challenging and developmental. But for counsellors early in their career one-to-one supervision is more supportive, as is having a supervisor from the same theoretical approach. Later in a career trying a supervisor from another approach is often an opportunity for personal and professional development, as the focus and style of supervision differs.

A further form of supervision arises in Randomised Controlled Trials and training for NICE approved interventions, such as Counselling for Depression and Cognitive Behavioural Therapy training for High Intensity IAPT workers. The task of the supervisor is to ensure that the counselling delivered sticks to the manualised treatment, that is, the supervisor must ensure adherence to the model. This is often done by listening to tape recordings of sessions and rating them for adherence with the model.

There are training courses in supervision offered in the three sectors that offer counselling training, but there is far greater diversity in supervision training than counsellor training. Universities and some of the Registered Awarding Organisations offer training in supervision. These courses last a year and in universities courses are postgraduate certificates and with Registered Awarding Organisations at Level 6. Usually students are required to be experienced counsellors in practice. In order to complete these courses students must also be working as supervisors and have supervision for the supervision they deliver. Supervision training in the private sector is very varied and may comprise only a few days (see Table 8.4).

It is not obligatory to have a qualification to work as a supervisor, and many supervisors have not undertaken formal training. It cannot be assumed that all counsellors will make good supervisors, as this is not the case.

Management of a counselling service

A second career path is a move into managing a counselling service. Counsellors working in services may take on different functions with experience, such as carrying out assessments, the allocation of clients to trainees and supervision. The move into managing a service represents a much bigger change, and in some cases a move into a different culture. There is no specific training for managing a counselling service. For some counsellors this may present the chance to blend together the skills and experiences from a first profession with counselling; for others it is more of a leap into the unknown.

There are many kinds of counselling services and therefore the scope of the management roles is great. The smallest change is a move to formal management of the clinical aspects of a counselling service. This might involve the oversight of initial client assessment, case allocation, case loads, management of the work of trainees and volunteers and supervision. Other management jobs have wider briefs.

A manager of an Employee Assistance Programme delivered within a large local government department will have targets to meet. Such targets can include waiting list times, throughput of clients and the need to prove efficiency and efficacy through, for example, being able to correlate a reduction in sickness rates with counselling service take up. Such a manager might have to impose a session limit regardless of client need, and therefore have access to good referral services. Many services use outcome measures such as CORE and the manager may terminate a counsellor's contract if the outcome measures show poor client improvement.

A manager of a charitable voluntary agency is likely to be accountable to a Board of Trustees and perhaps to a funding organisation as well. The smaller the agency the more responsibilities the manager may have. The manager in the local government EAP does not have to look after such things as Human Resources issues, pay roll, lighting and heating, building insurance and accounts. The agency manager probably does have to do all of this. In addition, the manager will have to oversee the staff, often a 'mixed economy' of staff, some employed, some volunteers and some trainees. If the service takes trainees there will be a placement contract with the training provider. Some managers of voluntary agencies have discovered that it costs to take on trainees in terms of additional assessment of clients to identify those suitable for trainees, the provision of in-house supervision and training and the evaluation and reports required by the training agency. Moving into management is a steep learning curve for most counsellors. Two particular challenges are holding to the values of counselling in the management role and maintaining a counselling practice. When I became the manager of a university student services department, the head of an academic department advised me, that I as the manager, would have to give up practice sooner or later. He was speaking from experience and still missed his discipline. I dismissed this helpful comment, thinking it wouldn't apply to me. But in time it did.

Training

Counsellors may move into work as tutors on counselling courses. One counsellor was taken on by the course he trained on, not long after qualification. This is not unusual, especially in private training organisations. There are additional requirements for people teaching in the Further or Higher Education sectors. Since 2007 new entrants to the Further Education sector have had to undergo initial teacher training within the first year of teaching to become a licensed practitioner and a further Certificate within the first five years. Qualified Teacher Learning and Skills Sector status is achieved by taking a Diploma in the subject. In Higher Education it is often compulsory for new staff on permanent contracts to have a postgraduate teaching qualification. These qualifications are often run in modular form by universities and are accredited by the Higher Education Association. Private training providers have their own selection criteria for staff. Tutor jobs in all of these sectors tend to be part time.

Voluntary work with the professional association

Another option for professional development is to become involved in the work of the professional association to which the counsellor belongs. Professional associations have many sections and interest groups made up of members, many also have open elections to the governing body. These are not jobs and will pay only expenses, but they open up huge networks, as well as providing limitless opportunities for development. Members are active in shaping the future of counselling. Members who become engaged in this way make friends who last a lifetime. This kind of voluntary activity can also lead to career opportunities, as the networks are large and people tend to think about whom they know when an opportunity arises. When I joined BACP as a student member, I had no idea that one day I would end up working full time for the association.

Snapshot of jobs available

To add substance to the previous sections, Table 8.5 provides a summary of the jobs advertised in one month in BACP's online jobs listing, followed by more details about the specific vacancies.

Table 8.5 *Examples of jobs available by sector in one month in 2013*

Sector/client group	Total
Children/young people	8
University	3
Primary Care/IAPT	5
Telephone counselling	1
Voluntary agency	3
Supervision	1
Training	2
Women refugees	3

Below are examples of jobs advertised in one month in 2013 in BACP's jobs online. They are set out by sector and career role, that is counsellor, supervisor, manager.

Health   The first two examples below show how different jobs with the same title can be.

1 Primary Care Counsellor, full time, Agenda for Change Band 6. Should be BACP accredited or accreditable.
2 Primary Care Counsellor, preferably self-employed. Should be accredited with BACP, CPC, UKCP or HCPC registered. The job will be brief therapy of 6–8 sessions, seeing 6 clients in an 8 hour day. Salary negotiable.
3 Psychosexual counsellor. £36,917–£46,837. Part time 8 hours a week to include life style counselling, health advice and specific therapies.
4 Eating Disorders Service Psychotherapists. £18.50 per hour for 10 clients a week over 2 to 3 days. £12 per hour for attendance at weekly service meetings. Counselling diploma or equivalent.

Children and young people

1 Upper school counsellor £21,516–£25,102. Full time, 1–6 pm term time on school premises. 12–14 hours a week client contact hours.
2 Sessional counsellor for primary school children £20.50 per hour. BACP accredited now or in next 6 months.

Employee assistance programme

1 Telephone counsellors. £20,600 pro rata, 24 hours a week includes weekends. To deliver brief focused therapy.

Voluntary sector counsellors

1 MIND volunteer counsellors. Must have a certificate in counselling and be in second year of a diploma/BSc/MSc. Must have had 50 hours of client work and be in personal therapy. To deliver short-term therapy. Also looking for qualified counsellors seeking experience.
2 Counsellor/psychotherapist for female refugees and asylum seekers. £17,383. 22 hours a week. Formal accredited training and qualification in counselling supervision.

Training

1 Training coordinator £5,090–£7,800. £15 per hour, 7–10 hours a week.

Voluntary sector posts with managerial or clinical responsibility

1   Counselling assessor pro rata £14,098–£15,754 21 hours a week. To manage referral and conduct one to one assessments.
2   Substance misuse counselling coordinator. £22,450–£28,070 Full time. Supervision of volunteers and placement students and have own caseload. BACP accredited and qualified supervisor.
3   Womens' project manager. £28,771–£30,351. Full time, women only. Should have a postgraduate qualification, three years' post qualifying experience and be accredited.
4   Place2Be School Project Manager. £24,814 pro rata 2 days a week. Manage a counselling service in a primary school and supervise Place2Be volunteers. Must have a recognised counselling or psychotherapy qualification.

Public sector managerial roles

1   University Head of Student Counselling. £50,570–£58,030 Full time. First degree and counselling qualification. BACP accreditation or UKCP registration or equivalent.

This list shows that there are jobs for counsellors, but these are likely to be part time and most are not very well paid. In November 2012 average annual earnings for full-time workers in the UK was £26,500 (BBC 2012). Only the jobs tied to Agenda for Change and the Head of the University Counselling Service reached or exceeded this figure.

CONCLUSION

It is to be hoped that the new model of professional quality assurance through the AVR scheme will make irrelevant the destructive rivalry within counselling and psychotherapy. There is no limit on the number of registers to be approved, as long as they meet the standards. Potentially it is a Dodo bird future where 'All shall win and all shall have prizes' (Lewis Carroll, quoted in Wampold 2001).

There is career progression for counsellors into management, supervision or training. In most of these posts counsellors are also expected to retain a small caseload. As said, this can become a challenge, especially in management positions. There is no obligation to develop a career path that moves away from work with clients. Many counsellors develop by specialising in work with a specific client group, such as eating disorders, or refugees, as the job advertisements show. What is important is to develop a career that satisfies you.

Counselling 'is a cultural invention that has made a huge contribution to the quality of life of millions of people' (McLeod 2009: 1–2). Counselling is a profession, counsellors work autonomously with complexity and the unknown. They balance conflicting ethical imperatives in the best interest of the client, given the imperfect knowledge with which they have to work. Often they do not know the outcomes of the work they do. Did the client improve or think counselling was a waste of time? They tend to be paid relatively little for what they do and have to hold several different jobs to make a living, or depend on income for non-counselling activities. Counsellors can never sit back complacent; they have an ethical requirement to present client work in supervision and strive to enhance their effectiveness and personal development. Counselling is not an easy job; professional relationship building with multiple people in distress, day in, day out is demanding. Finally in spite of, or perhaps because of all of the above, IT IS THE BEST JOB THERE IS.

REFERENCES

AGCAS (2012). *Prospects*. Available at www.prospects.ac.uk

Aldridge S. (2010). *Counselling – An Insecure Profession? A Sociological and Historical Analysis*. PhD. Leicester, University of Leicester.

Aldridge, S. and J. Pollard (2005). *Interim Report on the Mapping of Counselling and Psychotherapy*. London, Department of Health.

Aldridge, S., P. Coulter, et al. (2013). *Report on the BACP Adult Primary and Community Care Counselling Data Collection Exercise in Northern Ireland. (NI Demand and Capacity Model)*. Lutterworth, BACP.

BACP (2010). *Ethical Framework for Good Practice in Counselling and Psychotherapy*. Lutterworth, BACP.

BACP (2012). *Membership Survey*. Lutterworth, BACP.

Bond, T. (2010). *Standards and Ethics for Counselling in Action* (3rd edition). London, Sage.

Department for Children, Education, Lifelong Learning and Skills (2008). *School-based Counselling Services in Wales. A National Strategy*. Welsh Assembly Government.

Department of Education (2012). *Independent Counselling Service for Schools Handbook*. Northern Ireland Government.

Department of Health (2012). *Health and Social Care Act*. Department of Health.

Farsimadan, F., R. Draghi-Lorenz, et al. (2007). 'Process and outcome of therapy in ethnically similar and dissimilar therapeutic dyads.' *Psychotherapy Research* **17**(5): 567–75.

Government Social Research (2011). *Evaluation of the Welsh School-based Counselling Strategy. Final Report*. Welsh Assembly Government.

House, R. and N. Totton (Eds) (1997). *Implausible Professions. Arguments for Pluralism an Autonomy in Psychotherapy and Counselling*. Ross on Wye, PCCS Books.

Mann, R. (2006). *Workforce Development Study*. Rugby, BACP on behalf of the Qualification and Curriculum Authority.

McLaughlin, C., C. Holliday et al. (2013). *Research on Counselling and Psychotherapy with Children and Young People: A Systematic Scoping Review of the Evidence for the Effectiveness from 2003–2011*. Lutterworth, BACP.

McLeod, J. (2009). *An Introduction to Counselling*. Maidenhead, McGrawHill/Open University Press.

Moodley, R. (2007). 'Placing multiculturalism in counselling and psychotherapy.' *British Journal of Guidance and Counselling* **35**(1): 1–22.

Scaife, J. (2009). *Supervision in Clinical Practice: A Practitioner's Guide*. Hove, Routledge.

Symons, C. (2012). *Complaints and Complaining in Counselling and Psychotherapy: Organisational and Client Perspectives*. PhD. Leicester, University of Leicester.

Wampold, B. E. (2001). *The Great Psychotherapy Debate. Models, Methods and Findings*. London, Routledge.

Wheeler, S. and K. Richards (2007). *The Impact of Clinical Supervision on Counsellors and Therapists, their Practice and their Clients: A Systematic Review of the Literature*. Lutterworth, BACP.

INDEX

Page references to Figures or Tables will be in *italics*